Midwife Marley's Guide for Everyone

PREGNANCY, BIRTH & THE 4TH TRIMESTER

BLOOMSBURY PUBLISHING

LONDON · OXFORD · NEW YORK · NEW DELHI · SYDNEY

This book is dedicated to those
who have had a huge positive impact on
my life. Mum, you shaped me into the person
I am today, and for that I'm eternally grateful.
Tyrone, my soulmate – your continued love,
encouragement and support never go unnoticed.
To my children: you have taught me so much and
continue to do so. I love you all to the ends of
the Earth. Dad, if you were still with us, I know
you would be bursting with pride.
Miss you always.

Contents

About This Guide

Thank you for deciding to read my guide to pregnancy, birth and the fourth trimester. I have written this to help ease your journey from pregnancy to parenthood, using my experience as a midwife who has supported over 650 women through birth, and thousands more through their pregnancy and postnatal period.

As a mother of five children, including twins, I have also sat on the other side of the fence: the side you may be on right now, trying to anticipate the unknown and embarking on one of the most exciting journeys of your life. You may have lots of questions; not just about what happens while you're pregnant and during the birth, but also in the first few months after you have had your baby. As an eighteen-year-old having my first child, it would have helped me massively if I had known what to expect from life with a newborn prior to him being born. I managed to muddle my way through with guidance from my mother, but having an easy-to-read book I could refer to quickly through what felt like a never-ending cycle of feeding, changing and crying would have been a lifesaver. So, here it is, the book I wish I'd had for myself back then.

This guide is also a useful refresher for those who are expecting a subsequent child. From experience, sometimes it's easy to forget the journey and, of course, all pregnancies are different, so you may experience something new.

The guide is organised into three chapters, from pregnancy, to birth, to the fourth trimester and postnatal recovery. (If you haven't heard of the term 'fourth trimester' and are wondering what it means, it's the 3-6-month period after the baby is born.) Each chapter is divided into smaller sections to make it easier for you to find relevant information quickly – and bookmark sections that you want to catch up on later.

It might be an idea to get your birth partner to have a little read too; there is a section just for them on pages 160–163. They're likely to find the birth chapter particularly useful too, as the experience will be much more empowering if you both know what to expect.

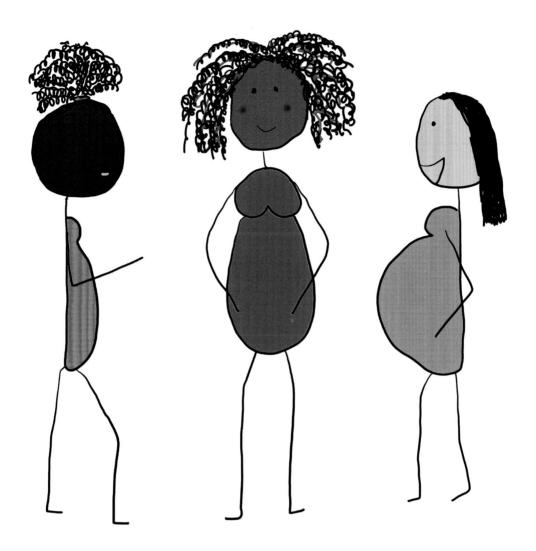

Babies are welcomed by parents from a diverse range of situations, as well as from a variety of cultural and ethnic backgrounds, making every experience unique. This guide is designed to be inclusive for absolutely all new and prospective parents, whether you are with a partner or not, in a same-sex relationship, or having a baby through surrogacy or adoption. I hope you enjoy reading it as much as I've enjoyed writing it!

Pregnancy

In This Chapter

So ... you've recently discovered you're pregnant. Congratulations!

The next 9 months or so will certainly be a journey for you and your family, one which may be filled with a range of emotions and feelings, from excitement, joy and energy to nausea, fatigue and learning to adjust to an ever-changing body. You may have recently carried out a home pregnancy test or had confirmation from your doctor that you are pregnant.

You may have suspected pregnancy, especially if you had been actively trying to conceive or have been experiencing early pregnancy symptoms, or this may just be a complete surprise. Either way, the first thing you'll want to do is think about your antenatal care. Your midwife will be able to provide you with information on what National Health Service (NHS) maternity services are available to you (you can access your midwife via your GP). Alternatively, you may want to seek care from an independent midwife instead, in which case Independent Midwives UK (*IMUK.org.uk*) is the place to go.

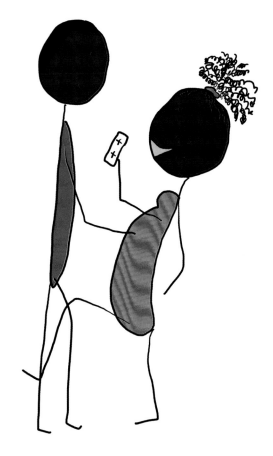

Due Dates

We mark '40 weeks' in our diary and imprint it in our brains like we have never marked anything before! Then we start the countdown.

It's sometimes hard to remember that the 'due date' is simply an estimate. Each time you visit your midwife, they will note down how many weeks' pregnant you are - the period of time you are pregnant is also referred to as 'gestation'.

On average, women are pregnant for 40 weeks, but it's not common for a woman to give birth on her due date. In fact, only 3-5 per cent of people give birth on their due date, with the majority having their babies in the week before or after. For women who go into labour naturally, most are born between 39 weeks and 41 weeks (plus 6 days' gestation).

Here are some gestation stats, from a survey I conducted on Instagram, that indicate the variation in lengths of pregnancy. I asked my followers how long their pregnancy was and over 3,000 women responded (the chart only includes stats for those who went into labour naturally, not planned caesareans or induced labours).

Gestation	Per cent of babies born then
under 35 weeks	2%
35 weeks–36 weeks + 6 days	7.5%
36 weeks–36 weeks + 6 days	5.8%
37 weeks–37 weeks + 6 days	10.6%
38 weeks–38 weeks + 6 days	12.7%
39 weeks–39 weeks + 6 days	16.2%
40 weeks–40 weeks + 6 days	21.9%
41 weeks–41 weeks + 6 days	18.6%
42 weeks–42 weeks + 6 days	3.5%
over 43 weeks	1.2%

So, you are likely to go into labour around your due date but not on it. I think we should start calling it a 'due window' instead!

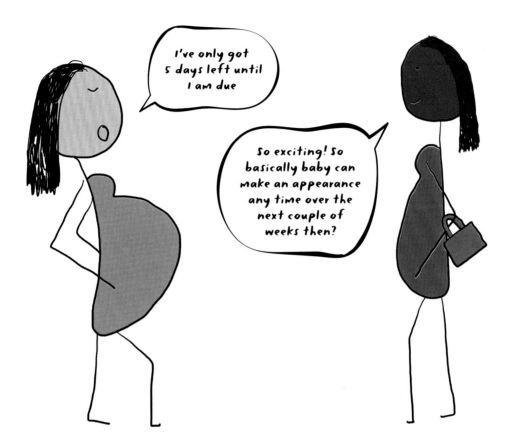

I've only got 5 days left until I am due

So exciting! So basically baby can make an appearance any time over the next couple of weeks then?

Your baby is likely to make an appearance any time between 37 and 42 weeks, so remember that before making too many plans!

One other thing to consider is that unless you have had assisted conception such as IVF (in vitro fertilisation), you won't know exactly when your date of conception is, even if you know when you had sexual intercourse. This is because sperm can live in the fallopian tubes and uterus for up to a week, therefore having sex a few days ago can result in conception when ovulation occurs today. Fascinating, right? So, because we don't know exactly when conception is, we count 9 months and 1 week (or 40 weeks) from the start day of your most recent period.

When you go for your first ultrasound scan, this date may be adjusted for accuracy, but even so, it is still an estimate. Babies will come when they are ready!

The Role Of Midwives And Doctors

During your pregnancy, birth and the postnatal period, you will encounter a number of health professionals who are there to support you and help plan your care. In the UK the system is fairly easy to understand and access, as we have the NHS. The main professionals that you will be likely to encounter are midwives and doctors specialising in pregnancy and birth.

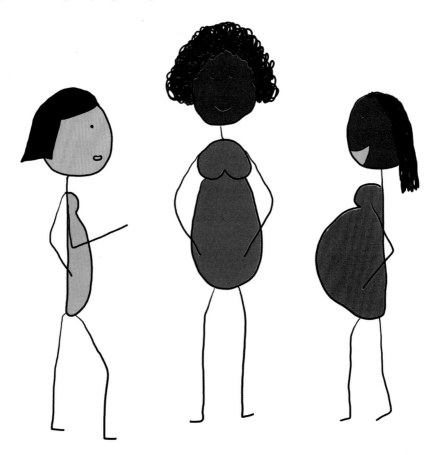

/ **MIDWIVES** have to be registered with the Nursing and Midwifery Council (NMC) in the UK to be able to practise in hospitals and birth centres up and down the country. Midwives are experts in physiological childbirth, having trained for several years at university and completed a number of clinical hours in a hospital setting. NHS midwives work in birth centres in hospitals and in the community, helping to bring babies into the world during birth, looking after them and their mothers on the wards, visiting new parents and their babies at home, and running antenatal clinics.

Midwives are great at identifying if things start to go off track, and referring someone to a doctor for additional care if need be. It is our role to provide evidence-based care and support mothers to make informed decisions around all aspects of their journey to parenthood. We like to use the term 'woman-centred' or 'client-centred' care, which is exactly what it should be!

/ **SPECIAL PREGNANCY DOCTORS**, called obstetricians or obstetric doctors, are experts in pregnancy and birth too. Obstetricians have trained for many years to become knowledgeable about childbirth and the complications that sometimes occur. In the UK they usually only become involved in a person's care if that person is deemed as having a 'complex' pregnancy (pages 18–19 discuss this further), or if an intervention is required in labour. Obstetricians are also skilled surgeons who can carry out caesareans and assisted births if necessary.

Midwives and doctors need to work closely together as a team to be able to provide optimal care for their clients during pregnancy, birth and beyond.

The NHS offers a 24/7 service to all, and is there for families throughout pregnancy, birth and postnatally. Some midwives and doctors work outside of the NHS in a private practice, however, and this can be appealing to those who prefer all their care to be with the same professional (which is not always guaranteed by the NHS). Private maternity hospitals provide full care with midwives and doctors for a cost. There are also private or independent midwives who can care for you through your pregnancy and birth if you choose to have a homebirth, though unless they are also employed by a hospital or birth centre, many independent midwives will not be able to assist at the actual birth for insurance reasons. (*IMUK.org* provides up-to-date information on this.)

If you opt for a private midwife to care for you throughout pregnancy and the postnatal period, you are still entitled to give birth in an NHS facility and have access to screening tests/ultrasounds they offer. I have cared for many clients on a private basis who have also attended an NHS hospital for their routine appointments.

Any UK resident is entitled to choose to have their baby in an NHS hospital, in a birth centre or at home. It's worthwhile checking what facilities are available in your local area.

Antenatal Appointments

When you first discover you are pregnant, you may wonder what the next 9 months are going to look like for you in terms of appointments with the midwife and/or hospital. If you are pregnant in the UK, you will be seen by a health professional at various points to monitor the wellbeing of both you and your baby.

What happens at each antenatal appointment very much depends on your gestation and how you are on the day. Blood pressure and urine samples are usually checked every time.

From around 25 weeks' gestation, your midwife will begin to measure your womb height (fundal height) with a tape measure. She may also listen to the baby's heartbeat at some point in the second trimester. Straightforward pregnancies are usually monitored by a midwife from booking right through to the birth, but you may not always see the same midwife. Some maternity units or birth centres are able to offer continuity of care – seeing the same midwife as much as possible – but with others it is less likely.

People who are classed as having a complex pregnancy (see pages 18–19) may find that they see a doctor as well as a midwife, and may have extra appointments for blood tests or scans, depending on their specific needs.

As a general rule, however, the schedule for antenatal appointments is as follows:

- 8–10 weeks
- 12 weeks (ultrasound)
- 16 weeks
- 20 weeks (ultrasound)
- 25 weeks (for first-time parents)
- 28 weeks
- 31 weeks (for first-time parents)
- 34 weeks, 36 weeks, 38 weeks, 40 weeks, 41 weeks

Antenatal appointments are the perfect time to ask questions and raise any concerns you may have.

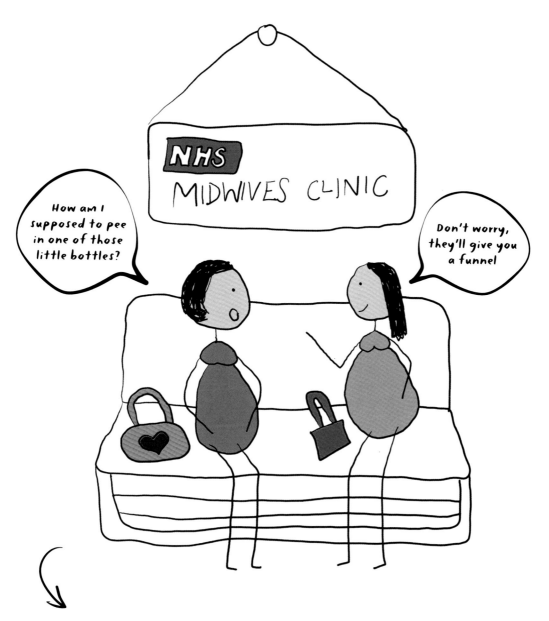

Write down any questions you have prior to going for your appointment - it will save you from forgetting.

Complex Or Straightforward Pregnancies

What factors can potentially make your pregnancy more complex?

During any stage of pregnancy, you may be told that your pregnancy is 'complex' ('high risk'). This term may sound a little scary, but it doesn't necessarily mean that problems will occur, it simply means that there are certain factors that may potentially cause complications in your pregnancy or labour, and health professionals may offer additional monitoring and care to prevent any problems arising. The majority of people who are considered to have 'complex' pregnancies for whatever reason actually go on to have uncomplicated pregnancies and births.

A woman who has a straightforward (low risk) pregnancy will usually have what is called 'midwife-led' care. She will see the midwife at various intervals throughout pregnancy and then be cared for during labour and birth by a midwife. Someone whose pregnancy is considered complex will usually be seen by both a midwife and obstetrician, often with both being involved during the labour and birth in one way or another.

When you have your initial booking appointment with the midwife, they will go through your medical history with you, making a number of assessments to determine if you are deemed to have a complex pregnancy or not. A complex pregnancy may require a different plan of care that includes visiting a number of other professionals, depending on your specific needs.

A few of the reasons a pregnancy may be considered 'complex' include:

- Pre-existing diabetes.
- Pre-existing high blood pressure.
- Pre-existing heart disease.
- Thyroid problems.
- Carrying more than one baby.
- Drug or alcohol dependence.
- Being significantly overweight or underweight.
- Age over 40.
- Age under 18.
- Previous caesarean.
- Previous preterm birth.
- Previous postpartum haemorrhage.
- Cervical surgery.
- Female genital mutilation.
- HIV.

Sometimes a pregnancy becomes complex as it progresses, and some of the reasons this can happen are due to:

- Pre-eclampsia.
- Placenta praevia.
- Placental insufficiency.
- Gestational diabetes.
- Obstetric cholestasis.

Being classed as having a complex pregnancy doesn't always place limitations on your birth, but it allows for closer monitoring, advice and sometimes treatment to ensure the safety of both you and your baby. As an example, a pregnancy that is complicated with a placenta praevia (a placenta that lies extremely close to the cervix, potentially obstructing the exit for the baby), may require additional ultrasounds throughout. If, by the end of the pregnancy, the placenta remains in its position, blocking the cervix, a caesarean may be advised.

Another example is having a baby over the age of 40. While there is a slight increase in the risk of complications such as pre-eclampsia, high blood pressure and placental problems, it's important to note that the majority of pregnancies at this stage are healthy and most women are able to give birth without complications.

Trimesters
Of Pregnancy

Pregnancies are divided into three trimesters, with each marking significant phases of development.

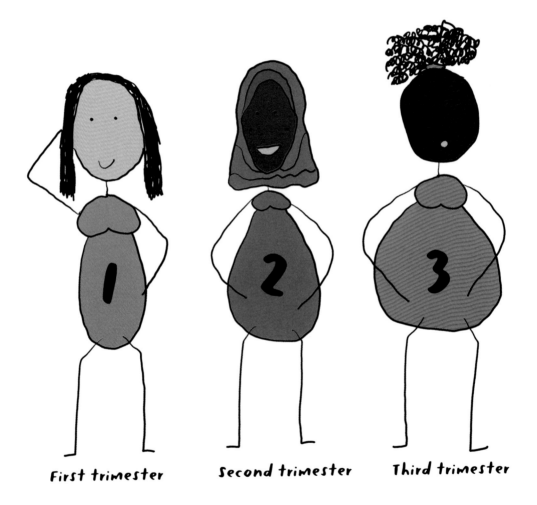

First trimester   Second trimester   Third trimester

First trimester

During the first trimester (up to **12 WEEKS**), your baby will go through a tremendous amount of developmental change, rapidly growing from a few cells to a visibly obvious human. Your baby will spend the next couple of trimesters growing, gaining weight and fine-tuning the development of their major organs. The first trimester is pretty tough for some women, as the fluctuation in pregnancy hormones can cause nausea, also known as 'morning sickness' (see pages 30–31). Other symptoms such as aversion to certain foods, breast tenderness, mood swings, strange tastes in your mouth, fatigue, and a change in sense of smell can be common during the first trimester too. During this time, you should have had an initial appointment with a midwife or doctor called the 'booking appointment'.

Second trimester

The second trimester starts at **13 WEEKS** and is the stage when many women find that their early pregnancy symptoms such as nausea have started to ease. Your baby is now growing rapidly and is moving lots in the womb. You may not be able to feel this until around 16–22 weeks, but some women feel it sooner, especially if they have had a baby before. The baby's genitals are usually identifiable on ultrasound by around 16–17 weeks, so if you want to find out the sex of the baby, you can ask at your 20-week 'anomaly scan'. You may find that your clothes are beginning to feel tight at the start of the second trimester or you may not! Everyone is individual and some 'show' earlier than others.

Third trimester

By the time the third trimester starts at **28 WEEKS**, your baby has developed into an amazing little person! They are quite active now and you should be feeling movements regularly each day. They spend their time gulping amniotic fluid (the liquid that surrounds the baby) in the womb and peeing it out again, and sometimes suck their thumbs to practise feeding and for comfort. They can also recognise your voice when you speak. You may find that your baby is very active at night when you are resting, as you are not walking around rocking them to sleep!

A lot of brain and lung development needs to occur between 28 and 40 weeks. Although a baby born at 28 weeks has a good chance of survival with neonatal intensive care, a baby born closer to 40 weeks will be less likely to need any interventions. The last few weeks of your pregnancy will feel tiring due to carrying your rapidly growing baby, you may find that you are constantly running to pee, and the baby's head may put pressure on your pelvic floor, making it difficult to walk without waddling! This stage is the home straight and it won't be long before you're holding your baby in your arms.

"

Only 3–5 per cent of people give birth on their due date, with the majority having their babies in the week before or after.

"

Having A Healthy Pregnancy

Remaining as healthy as possible will not only help to promote the best environment for your growing baby, it will also keep you feeling good too.

Diet and supplements

I bet you've heard enough old wives' tales surrounding eating in pregnancy to last you a lifetime, right? Well, most old wives' tales are just that: tales! It is important, however, to have a balanced, healthy diet to ensure your baby's optimum growth and development and help you feel as good as you possibly can during this time. Pregnancy can take its toll if you are lacking in vitamins and minerals, as the baby will draw everything they need from you, leaving you feeling drained.

In general it's best to get vitamins and minerals from the foods you eat rather than from supplements, as they are absorbed more easily, but during pregnancy it's advised to take an extra folic acid supplement as well, to help prevent neural tube defects such as spina bifida developing in the baby. Most of us eating a Western diet don't consume the recommended amount of foods containing folic acid, such as leafy greens and chickpeas, hence why supplements are advised. Although it's not usually required, if you decide you would like to take multi-vitamin supplements during pregnancy, avoid any containing vitamin A, as high amounts can cause birth defects. Also, avoid high-dose vitamins, and if in doubt, stick to ones that are labelled as suitable for pregnancy.

Having a balanced diet means making sure you eat a varied selection of:

- Fruit and vegetables.
- Carbohydrates (pasta, rice, potatoes).
- Protein (beans, pulses, fish, eggs, poultry).

Aim to eat at least five portions of fruit and veg each day, and remember to wash fresh produce before consumption. Processed fruit juices (such as many cartons of juice) should be avoided, as they often contain a lot of sugar. Opt for fresh juice instead.

Where possible, try to choose lean meat and ensure all meat is cooked thoroughly, with no pink meat, and that the meat juices run clear.

Drinking plenty of water during pregnancy is important to prevent dehydration. It is recommended you drink 1.5–2 litres of water per day (six to eight average glasses).

Cravings

Pregnancy cravings can be the strangest thing, and they are not limited to foods (as many may think) – craving smells is also pretty common. Some people have no cravings at all (it's different for each person), but if you do, they usually start in the first trimester. They tend to intensify in the second trimester and in the third trimester you might find cravings stop.

Some women will crave fatty foods like chips or cake, some may long for foods that don't usually go together such as pickles and chocolate, and some can't get enough of the smell of onions. Try to eat as healthily as you can, even though the temptations to gorge on certain foods may be strong!

Often women will feel an overwhelming urge to eat non-food items. This is called 'pica' and it can lead to you wanting to eat things such as chalk, dirt, ashes, coffee grounds, laundry detergent, clay and more. The causes of pica are not well understood, though some studies suggest that it's linked to a mineral deficiency, most commonly of iron.

Depending on what non-food items you're craving, pica may be dangerous both to you and to the baby. Eating things like dirt, ash and clay can damage and even obstruct your digestive tract, which can lead to serious infections. Craving ice chips (like I did) probably won't do any harm!

If you're having non-food cravings, you should speak to your doctor or midwife to determine if you have any underlying physical or mental health issues. You may need to take a blood test to ensure that you have healthy levels of iron and other necessary nutrients.

Foods and drink to avoid or consume with caution

Some foods put you at a greater risk of developing food poisoning – something that you particularly don't want when pregnant. Food poisoning can lead to miscarriage, preterm birth and even stillbirth, so it's best to be extra careful. Some drinks should also be avoided or limited. These are foods and drinks to avoid or be cautious about:

/ **OILY FISH**. When you're pregnant, avoid having more than two portions of oily fish such as salmon, trout, mackerel or herring per week. It can contain toxins which may be harmful if eaten in large quantities.

/ **RAW EGGS**. Avoid raw or partially cooked eggs as there is a risk of salmonella. Eggs produced under the British Lion Code of Practice, however, are safe for pregnant women to eat raw or partially cooked, as they come from chickens that have been vaccinated against salmonella. These eggs have a red lion logo stamped on their shell.

/ **SOFT CHEESE**. Soft cheeses that have been pasteurised such as cottage cheese, mozzarella, feta, cream cheese, paneer, ricotta, halloumi, goats' cheese without a rind (white coating on the outside) and processed cheese spreads are okay to eat. Soft cheeses such as Brie, Camembert and chèvre, and soft blue cheeses such as Danish blue, Gorgonzola and Roquefort can be eaten if they are cooked thoroughly. They should be steaming-hot throughout to ensure any bacteria has been killed. All unpasteurised milk and unpasteurised milk products should be avoided due to the risk of listeria. (Listeria can lead to listeriosis which has been linked to miscarriage and stillbirth.)

/ **ALCOHOL** should be avoided during pregnancy as there are no 'safe amounts' currently recognised by the Department of Health in the UK.

/ **CAFFEINE** should be limited to 200mg (one to two mugs of coffee or three to four mugs of tea) per day.

Exercise

Did you just roll your eyes? It's okay – when I was told how important exercise is during pregnancy when I was having my first child I did too. If you are someone who exercises regularly anyway, keep it up as long as you feel comfortable. Exercise is not dangerous for your baby and there is actually some evidence to suggest that keeping fit can help reduce the likelihood of complications later on in pregnancy and during labour. One Spanish study* concluded that women who were regularly exercising during pregnancy had slightly shorter labours, so it's worth keeping active!

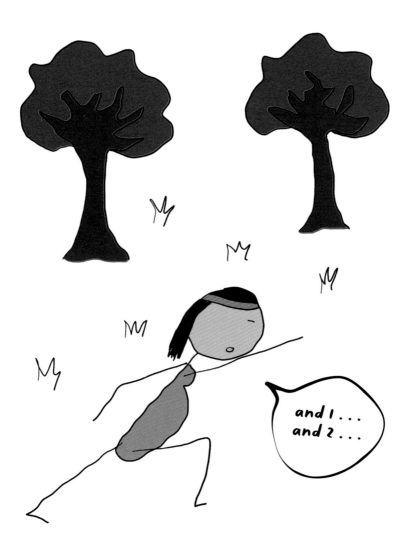

If you don't find exercise particularly thrilling, even a simple 15–20-minute walk to the shops is beneficial. If you don't fancy the walk (perhaps you're pregnant in winter and it's cold), take the stairs if you have them. Walking up and down your stairs a few times a day is a great cardio activity and also gets those muscles toned, which is all-important for the big day.

Most moderately strenuous sports are okay if you are used to doing them pre-pregnancy. For example, if you enjoyed weight-lifting pre-pregnancy, you can continue for as long as you feel comfortable. However it's not a good idea to start any new sports, other than light ones such as swimming and yoga, during pregnancy.

Smoking

If you smoke, you will be well aware that it isn't easy to quit. It is, however, very important to cut out smoking during pregnancy to ensure the healthy development of your baby.

There are over 4,000 chemicals in each cigarette which can affect your baby. Smoking also restricts the amount of oxygen that your baby receives, often causing growth restriction.

Speak to your midwife about the NHS smoking cessation service or visit nhs.uk/pregnancy/keeping-well/stop-smoking for more support.

Recreational drug use

It can be really tough to stop using illegal or recreational drugs, however suddenly stopping can also be unsafe for you and your baby. If drug use is something you struggle with, it's important that you speak to your doctor or midwife so that you can get all the help and support you need. The effect drugs have on your pregnancy will depend on the type and quantities taken, along with your general health.

It may feel pretty daunting speaking openly about drug addiction, and many expectant women will fear the reaction of their care provider. Be assured though that all they will want to do is to help you overcome your addiction to encourage the best health of you and your baby.

*SOURCE: BARAKAT R, FRANCO E, PERALES M, LÓPEZ C, MOTTOLA MF. EXERCISE DURING PREGNANCY IS ASSOCIATED WITH A SHORTER DURATION OF LABOR. A RANDOMIZED CLINICAL TRIAL. EUR J OBSTET GYNECOL REPROD BIOL. 2018 MAY;224:33-40. DOI: 10.1016/J.EJOGRB.2018.03.009. EPUB 2018 MAR 6. PMID: 29529475.

Spotting During Pregnancy

'Spotting' during pregnancy refers to a small amount of blood-stained discharge, which you may notice in your underwear, or when you wipe after going to the toilet.

Spotting is certainly a scary thing for a pregnant woman to see. If you have previously suffered a pregnancy loss it's even more so, and you may find yourself running to the bathroom to check for bleeding multiple times throughout the day, but it does not always mean there is a problem with the pregnancy.

Most of the time spotting is brown or pink and occurs in the first trimester. It is often associated with something called 'implantation bleeding'. This is spotting that occurs extremely early in pregnancy at the time when the fertilised egg implants into the lining of the uterus, causing it to shed a little. It doesn't happen to everyone but it is fairly common. Implantation bleeding is more likely to occur 6–12 days after conception, which is often the time when you would expect a period. This can be confusing to some people, as they may mistake this spotting for an extremely light period.

If you have recently had sexual intercourse or have an infection in the vagina or cervix, this can cause irritation and spotting too. In these instances, call your care provider for further advice.

If you ever experience any bright-red persistent bleeding, with or without pain, at any stage during your pregnancy, always contact your care provider without delay.

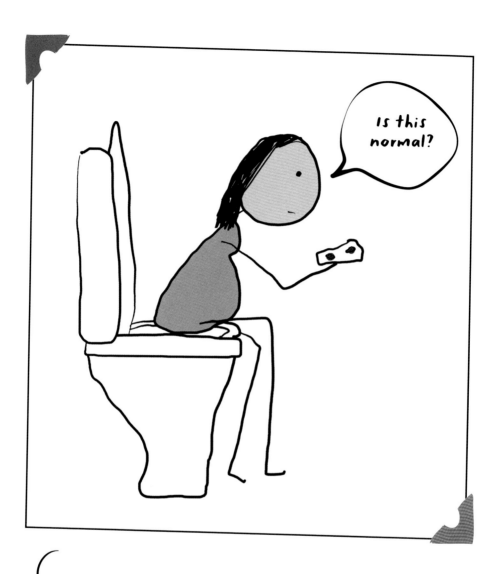

Many women (about one in five) will experience some form of spotting during their pregnancy.

Nausea And Vomiting

Nausea and vomiting in pregnancy is often referred to as 'morning sickness'. This should actually be called 'anytime sickness' as it doesn't just occur in the morning!

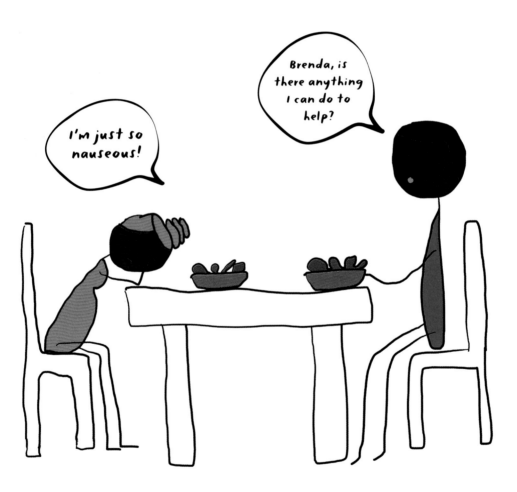

Nausea and/or vomiting in pregnancy is not nice at all for those who suffer from it. Some women will experience mild symptoms, some experience severe symptoms, and some will be fortunate enough to escape it altogether. Some women will find the nausea and/or vomiting disappears by the second trimester, and some will suffer throughout pregnancy. One big factor is hormones, specifically the HCG (pregnancy hormone) levels – the higher they are, the more likely you will suffer with the dreaded nausea, and HCG levels usually peak by the end of the first trimester.

Finding effective methods for alleviating nausea is a personal thing. For some women nothing works, and they find themselves asking the doctor for medication to help. For others, doing simple things like eating small meals often, avoiding strong smells, avoiding fatty/spicy foods and having a dry snack on the bedside table for when they wake might help. Some women just feel nauseous and others will also vomit.

Severe morning sickness is called Hyperemesis gravidarum (HG) and it causes pregnant women to vomit multiple times per day. Hyperemesis gravidarum is a debilitating form of vomiting in pregnancy that affects around 1 per cent of pregnancies. Experiencing nausea and vomiting persistently and severely day and night can really take its toll, emotionally and physically. The most common symptoms of HG include:

- Constant nausea.
- Vomiting *at least* three to four times per day. Many people with HG will vomit at least twenty times daily.
- Feeling lightheaded and dizzy.
- Inability to keep down any food or fluid, which leads to dehydration.
- Loss of more than 5 per cent of your bodyweight due to the constant nausea and vomiting.

The likelihood of developing HG increases in the case of multiple pregnancies (twins/triplets etc.) and/or a family history of HG and trophoblastic disease, which causes an abnormally high level of cell growth within the uterus.

If you are suffering from continuous vomiting, it's crucial that you seek help from your care provider, as dehydration can set in quickly if you can't keep fluids down. For severe cases, admittance to hospital may be necessary, to be hydrated via a drip.

How HG is managed very much depends on the severity of symptoms and how it is affecting your pregnancy. Sometimes it can be managed with anti-emetics (anti-sickness medications) but each case is individual. HG very often lasts throughout pregnancy, although some recover after a couple of months.

Antenatal Blood Tests

At the first appointment with your midwife, they will offer to take a blood sample to check for various things such as your blood group, the presence of antibodies, iron levels, hepatitis and HIV status, random glucose levels and absence of syphilis. If you are from an ethnic group where inherited blood conditions sickle cell and thalassaemia are more prevalent, you may also be offered a test for these.

After the first appointment and blood test, further blood tests are offered at around 28 and 34 weeks, including a full blood count and antibody test. At 28 weeks there is also the option of another random glucose test.

Some women may also be offered a fasting glucose tolerance test which is different from the random one. The glucose tolerance test (GTT) determines how your body processes a large amount of sugar in a small timeframe after not eating anything for several hours. If it's deemed appropriate, it is routinely performed at 26–28 weeks of pregnancy (earlier if you have previously had gestational diabetes). Some people are more likely than others to develop gestational diabetes, if they have:

- A family history of diabetes.
- A body-mass index (BMI) greater than 30.
- Previously had a larger-than-average-weight baby.
- Previously had gestational diabetes.
- A Black, South Asian or Middle Eastern family background.

The test itself involves drinking a carefully-measured glucose drink, followed two hours later by a blood test to check your blood sugar levels. If you are offered one of these tests, you should be given instructions on when to stop eating prior to the test – it's usually midnight before, so make sure you have a decent meal as late as you can, as you might be hungry in the morning!

If the result comes back indicating glucose intolerance, you may be referred for further investigations and will most likely be under the care of a diabetic specialist midwife.

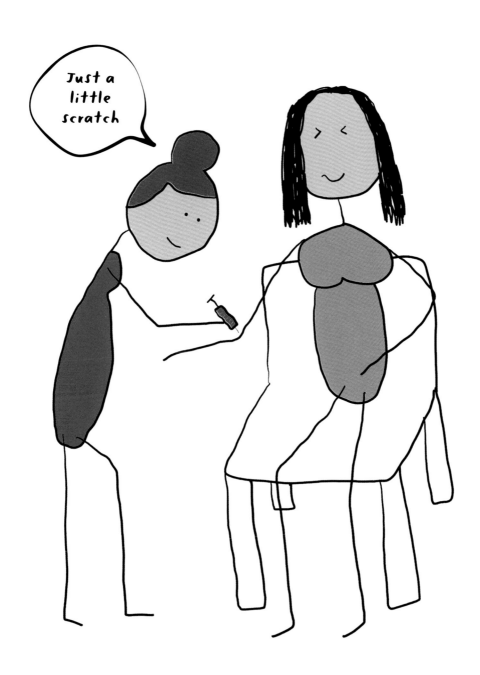

Ultrasound Scans

You can expect to be offered two routine ultrasound scans during pregnancy: one at 10-14 weeks and one at 18-22 weeks.

The first ultrasound

The purpose of the first ultrasound scan at 10-14 weeks is to confirm your gestation and to check on the wellbeing of the baby. This ultrasound takes 20-30 minutes to complete. A screening test called the 'combined test' is also offered at the first ultrasound to calculate your chance of having a baby with Down's syndrome, along with a couple of other rare congenital disorders, including Patau's and Edwards' syndromes. This involves taking a blood sample to look for certain markers that may indicate a higher chance of having a baby with one of these disorders. Your midwife or doctor will discuss this test with you prior to having the ultrasound and blood test. It's important to remember that this is not a diagnostic test, it just gives you a risk factor which estimates the likelihood of having a baby with these congenital disorders. If the results of the test show you have a higher likelihood than most, you will be offered further testing.

The second ultrasound

The second ultrasound you are offered, at 18-22 weeks, is called the 'anomaly scan'. It's a detailed ultrasound which checks the baby's growth and all of their major organs to make sure everything is as it should be. This ultrasound usually takes thirty to forty minutes.

If you have chosen to have the two routine ultrasound scans, there usually aren't any further scans unless there is an indication that more are needed, e.g. your midwife is concerned about the baby's growth.

Amniotic fluid levels are also measured during ultrasound scans. This will give an early warning if there is too much fluid around the baby (polyhydramnios) or too little fluid (oligohydramnios).

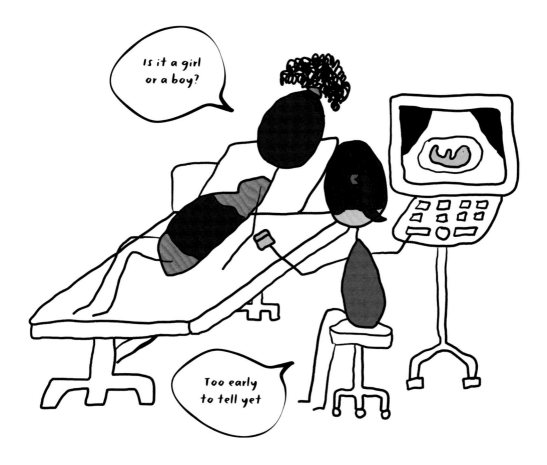

/ **POLYHYDRAMNIOS** affects around 2 per cent of pregnancies and is detected on ultrasound usually when a woman's fundus (top of the uterus) is measuring much larger than what is typical for her stage of pregnancy. Often the cause isn't clear, but it can be due to an abnormality with the baby, maternal diabetes, infection during pregnancy or blood incompatibility between mother and her baby. Complications can include preterm birth, early membrane rupture, cord prolapse and placental abruption. If you have polyhydramnios, your doctor will offer extra monitoring and potentially extra scans too.

/ **OLIGOHYDRAMNIOS** affects around 8 per cent of pregnancies and can be caused by many factors including preterm rupture of membranes, maternal issues such as pre-eclampsia, and kidney or urinary tract anomalies in the foetus. Oligohydramnios in the second half of pregnancy can cause growth restriction in babies and early birth. If you have oligohydramnios and are very preterm, you will be offered extra monitoring via ultrasound and CTG or non-stress tests. If close to your due date, you may be offered induction of labour.

Five things to consider before your ultrasound scans

1. **DISCUSS THE COMBINED TEST**
Discuss the combined test with your partner and midwife prior to going to the first ultrasound appointment. This will give you time to do research of your own, read any literature your midwife gives you, and decide if you want to have the test. You can opt out of the combined test if you wish, but can still have the ultrasound.

2. **YOU DON'T NEED A FULL BLADDER**
Don't make yourself needlessly uncomfortable by drinking too much fluid. Years ago, when the technology was less advanced, full bladders were essential for ultrasounds, so you may find friends and family members who gave birth over 15 years ago advising you to do this!

3. **MAKE SURE YOU HAVE EATEN SHORTLY BEFORE YOU GO FOR THE SCAN**
Avoid going hungry, or take a snack with you, as you may be in for a wait, especially afterwards with the combined blood test at the first scan.

4. **TAKE SOME CHANGE AND A DEBIT/CREDIT CARD**
Having money will be handy if you want to purchase a picture of your baby to take home.

5. **TRY TO AVOID TAKING CHILDREN WITH YOU**
Ultrasounds in pregnancy can be quite long and children do get restless!

NOTE: Ultrasound technology is a very useful way to assess the development of your baby, but it is not 100 per cent accurate at identifying the exact gestation or size/weight of the baby, and sometimes other diagnostic tests such as blood tests are required to pick up any potential issues.

RHD Incompatibility:
blood groups and Rh-negative blood

Knowing your blood group is important in pregnancy and is one of the things that is checked at your first appointment with your midwife.

The most common blood groups are A, B, AB and O. Your blood group is determined genetically at conception – it's a perfect combination of your parents' DNA! It's classified as A, B, AB or O based on an antigen (a type of protein marker) that is present on the cell. Now this is where it gets a little more complicated: after the letter, there is also a '+' or a '-' symbol. This is determined by blood-cell antigens, as well. If you are '+' (positive), it means that your blood cells carry the Rh (rhesus) antigen. If you are '-' (negative), there is no Rh antigen. In this instance you would be classed as rhesus-negative. As an example, if your blood is marked with the 'A' protein marker and also contains an Rh antigen, your blood type is A+. If your blood is marked with both 'A' and 'B' proteins but no Rh antigen is found, your blood type will be AB- and so on.

So, why is this so important to know? If someone needs a transfusion during or after pregnancy, a compatible blood type needs to be given. You will only know which blood is compatible by finding out your blood group. (A transfusion is a remote possibility for most people, and is only required in the event of a postpartum haemorrhage – see pages 156–157.)

The other reason it's important to know your blood type is down to Rh incompatibility. If a mother is rhesus negative (let's say she's A-) and the baby she's carrying is B+, because that's dad's blood group, there is a small chance the baby's blood might mix with the mother's. If this happens, the mother then starts to produce antibodies which can cause complications when the baby is born.

To avoid this, people who are rhesus negative are offered an injection of a blood product called Anti-D during pregnancy. Anti-D effectively neutralises any Rh-positive blood cells from the baby that have entered the mother's bloodstream before the body has a chance to start producing antibodies. Your midwife or doctor will tell you whether or not you are recommended to have the Anti-D injection once your initial blood group results are back.

Skin And Hair Changes

Skin and hair changes are super common in pregnancy, particularly in the early stages.

Normally, around 85–95 per cent of your hair is in the growth phase at any point in time, but hormonal changes during pregnancy stimulate an increase. As a result, many women enjoy thicker hair during pregnancy, as more hairs than normal are growing and fewer than normal are resting/shedding. You can read more about what happens to this hair afterwards on page 214. Skin changes can be pretty alarming, and spotty breakouts in pregnancy are common. These breakouts can tend to hit sometime in the first trimester – usually at around 6 weeks. Hormone surges (in this case progesterone, which causes your glands to increase acne-causing secretions of oil, called sebum) can clog up pores and cause bacteria to build up, leading to breakouts, and your body is also retaining more fluid which contains toxins that can lead to acne breakouts.

If you experience skin breakouts in pregnancy, be sure to keep your skin clean, and moisturise with an oil-free moisturiser to help with any discomfort and itchiness. For most women, as the pregnancy progresses the skin tends to clear up and it may even start to glow! Aside from spots, you may find that your skin becomes dry during pregnancy. This can be due to hormone changes causing your skin to lose elasticity and moisture as it stretches and tightens to accommodate a growing belly. Some women even report pigment changes, with their skin developing darker areas on the face. This is due to your body producing more melanin, a pigment which helps to protect your body from the sun's UV rays.

Breast changes may also be noticeable during pregnancy. You might find that they become more tender, the skin around the nipple (areola) may darken, veins may appear more prominent, and you may even notice colostrum, the first milk, leaking later on in the third trimester. If you don't, it's nothing to worry about. Comfort is key, so wear a well-fitted bra as you may find your breasts increase in size throughout pregnancy. You can wear underwired bras if they feel comfortable and give you more support. Many people ask me about wearing a bra to bed – if it helps support your breasts and feels comfortable for you then that's absolutely fine. You can read more about breastfeeding on pages 186–195.

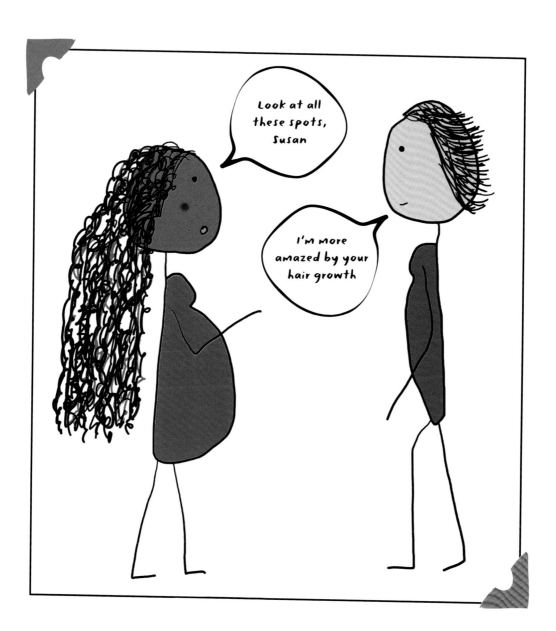

Emotional Changes

Hormones are responsible for a lot of changes in pregnancy, including emotional ups and downs. It's pretty common to feel like everything is making you tearful, or find that one minute you're laughing and the next you're crying!

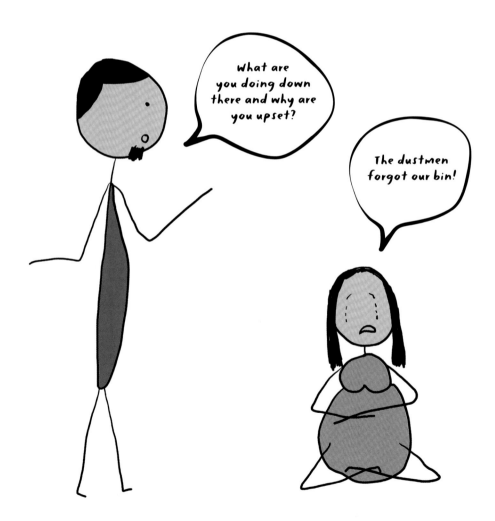

Sometimes, persistent low mood can be a sign of something a little more serious than emotional ups and downs. Antenatal depression is a change in mood that is persistent and more severe than the average tearfulness that a woman may experience a handful of times throughout pregnancy. Signs include:

- An unusual amount of worry about giving birth and parenthood.
- Lack of energy and disturbed sleep.
- Losing interest in yourself or your pregnancy.
- Feeling emotionally detached, teary, angry or irritable.
- Chronic anxiety.
- Poor concentration.
- Sense of hopelessness about the future.

You may not have all of these symptoms but if any of these become concerning, you should speak with your doctor or midwife.

There are events which occur in a person's life which can increase the likelihood of developing antenatal depression such as: a history of depression, previous miscarriage, stillbirth or infant loss, previous traumatic birth, social factors such as isolation, domestic abuse, poverty, difficult childhood issues and low self-esteem. For some women, though, antenatal depression can just happen out of the blue with no known trigger.

Women who suffer antenatal depression are more likely to suffer postnatal depression too, which means it's important you share any concerns with someone so that help and support can be put in place. The best people to discuss this with are your GP, midwife, or organisations such as Tommy's and PANDAS Foundation (charities that help those struggling during and after pregnancy with mental health issues).

Sleep

'Sleep as much as you can now – you won't be able to when the baby arrives.' Sound familiar? I remember people saying that to me continually when I was pregnant with my first child. Only problem was, it wasn't that easy!

Trying to get a decent night's sleep when there is a huge bump in the way, your breasts are aching, and you're feeling nauseous, isn't as simple as it sounds. You may find that you suffer bouts of insomnia during pregnancy as you try to get into a comfortable sleeping position. This can be helped by placing a pillow between the knees and ensuring you have a relaxing downtime routine in the evening.

So, what about the sleeping position? You may have read or heard that sleeping flat on your back is not recommended during pregnancy. There is some truth to this, although it really only refers to when your bump is growing bigger – from around 16 weeks onwards. If you lie flat on your back to go to sleep, the entire weight of your uterus rests on your back, intestines and major blood vessels running from the heart. This pressure can subsequently aggravate backache, hinder digestion and interfere with optimal blood circulation. You may notice that if you lie flat when your midwife examines you at routine appointments, you feel a little dizzy after. This is because of the restricted blood flow caused by the uterus pressing on those blood vessels, affecting your blood pressure. This less-than-optimum circulation may also have an impact on the delivery of vital oxygen and nutrients to your baby.

Ideally, lying on your side during pregnancy to sleep is preferred, your left side if possible, as the major blood vessel runs along the right side. Either side, however, is better than your back. Don't panic if you wake up and you are flat on your back – just simply roll back onto your side. Most of us move around during sleep and will naturally get ourselves into the optimal position without even being conscious of it.

Lying on your belly is comfortable for many people, until they fall pregnant! You may find that you can sleep on your front up until you enter the second trimester when it becomes uncomfortable.

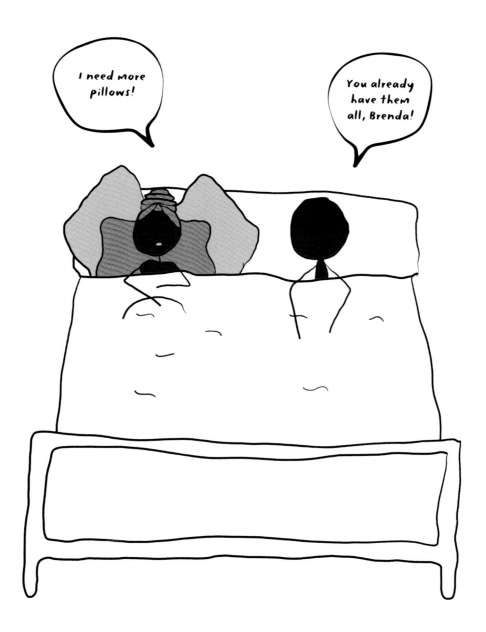

Relationships

Pregnancy, as natural as it is, can take its toll on you both physically and emotionally.

The sudden shift in hormone levels during pregnancy can often cause you to be more sensitive than usual. For example, you may find you cry more easily at things that would never usually upset you, and you may have less patience. This, coupled with external factors that some may experience such as future financial anxieties a baby may bring, or other practical stresses, can put a strain on close relationships. This isn't limited to partners; it can be your friends, parents, siblings, or anyone who is close to you. Often, though, it's the relationship with your partner that can be affected the most during pregnancy. It's common for couples to have disagreements, even in a healthy relationship.

Some of the common reasons that people argue during pregnancy include:

- You feel that you are more interested in the pregnancy than they are.
- You think your partner is being overprotective, e.g. not letting you lift things, or commenting on your diet.
- You both have anxieties about the financial and practical responsibility of becoming parents.
- One of you wants to have sex but the other doesn't.
- You feel nauseous, tired and moody.
- You feel self-conscious or insecure about your changing body and think your partner no longer finds you attractive.

When you have your first child as a couple, making that leap to parenthood isn't always an easy one. In fact it's one of the most life-changing events you can go through! It's a good idea to talk to each other about how you're feeling at present and any future anxieties you may have. Sometimes it's difficult to do this, especially if the conversation becomes negative or is filled with accusations. Having some time to yourself – perhaps going for a pamper session or out for dinner with friends – might help give you the space you may need before trying to resolve things again. There are times when talking about how you feel doesn't prevent arguing, but it can still help prepare you for the changes ahead and allow you to get things off your chest rather than building it all up and becoming frustrated.

Bump Size

Pregnant women come in all different shapes and sizes. Shorter women may appear to have bigger bumps compared to taller women; those with a little extra weight may appear bigger than those with slimmer frames; and first-time mums may have smaller bumps than women who have had a baby before.

The fundal height measurement (the measurement from the pubic bone to the top of the womb, not the top of your belly) is usually checked in the UK from 25 weeks to get an idea of how the uterus (and subsequently baby) is growing. It's not 100 per cent accurate so is only used as a guide.

Generally speaking, at 25 weeks' gestation, the fundal height will measure around 25cm, give or take a couple of centimetres each side. Each time you visit your midwife the measurement should increase by approximately 1cm per week. If there is any indication that the baby is not growing as they should be (i.e. the fundal height measurement hasn't changed from one appointment to the next, or is measuring much smaller than expected) you might be referred for an ultrasound. In most cases the growth scan turns out to be normal, but occasionally a problem may be noted with the placenta or there might be reduced amniotic fluid. If you measure overly big on the other hand, it may be because of higher than usual levels of fluid.

Measuring fundal height is not a useful indicator in all circumstances, however. The measurement will be different for women who are carrying twins, who have fibroids and those who have a very high BMI (Body Mass Index is a tool to calculate if your weight is healthy). Most of the time the size of your bump is fine, no matter how big or small you look on the outside.

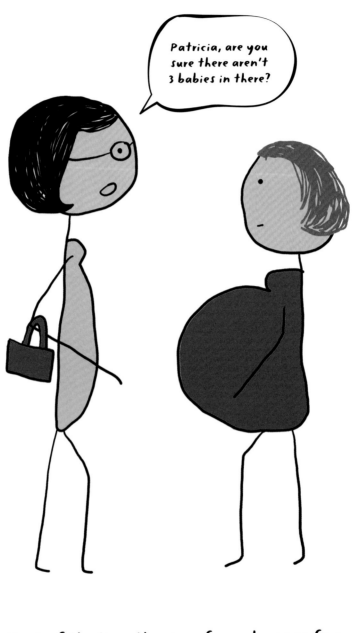

Most of the time the size of your bump is fine,
no matter how big or small you look on the outside.

Weight Gain During Pregnancy

Weight gain in pregnancy varies from woman to woman. Ultimately, it depends on how much you weigh before you become pregnant.

Most pregnant women gain 10–12.5kg, putting on most of the weight after week 20. This is just an average though, as some women put on less than this and many will put on more – like me, who puts on around 20kg each time!

Much of the extra weight is due to your baby growing, but your body will also be storing fat, preparing itself to make breastmilk after your baby is born. Water retention is also a factor in weight gain during pregnancy. As long as you are eating as sensibly as you can (not always easy when pregnant, I know!), then try not to worry too much.

If your care provider notes that your pre-pregnancy BMI is lower or higher than the recommended healthy range, you might be given some extra dietary advice and monitoring. The long-used BMI calculator isn't the most accurate tool in deciding if someone is under- or over-weight. It focuses on height and weight, not taking into consideration things like age, sex, ethnicity, bone density and general health. And it doesn't measure muscle mass either, so if you are a body builder, for example, you may find yourself having a higher BMI than someone who isn't.

Ethnicity plays a major role too. A black female with a BMI of 27 may be classed as slightly overweight according to the generalised BMI charts we see in the UK. However, people of African descent tend to have less visceral fat (fat around organs) and more muscle mass. As muscle is denser than fat, these standardised charts may see a black woman labelled as overweight or obese when she is not.

For Asian women, this cut-off for a healthy BMI is a lot lower than that for white women, so by using the standardised charts, we are potentially classing some women as having a healthy BMI when in fact they are overweight and missing out on extra monitoring and advice.

Pregnancy With A Toddler (Or Two)

Being pregnant and a mum is a lot different to being pregnant with your first baby, especially if your child is under four years old. You tend to feel much more tired and the opportunity to just go and have a nap often isn't there like it was the first time around!

Going through pregnancy when your eldest child is a toddler is something that many women have been through, as it's common to have an age gap of a couple of years between babies. You might be worried about how you will cope with lack of sleep, a boisterous toddler and even feelings of 'how will I manage to share the love between my eldest and my new baby?'.

You may be feeling burned out from juggling everything, especially if you are working too. I only experienced having a toddler while pregnant when I was carrying my fifth baby. Prior to that I had larger age gaps of 7 and 9 years. Having to care for a toddler, when you have a big bump and just want to rest, is demanding. My advice is, if your toddler is still napping, try to lie down and take a nap with them!

If you have the offer of support from others, accept help where possible. If you don't have much in the way of family support or friends locally, you might want to consider exploring the idea of a nursery or childminder, even if it's just for three or so hours a couple of days a week, so that you can recharge. If your child is at least 2 years old, you may be entitled to free childcare, depending on your circumstances. By the age of 3, all children in the UK are entitled to at least fifteen hours of free nursery childcare each week. For more information, see *childcarechoices.gov.uk*.

You may want to think ahead about the care of your child when you go into labour. If you're having a homebirth, is there someone who can come and keep your little one occupied if it's during the day? If you're intending on giving birth in a hospital or birth centre, it might be worth working out who will be supporting you with childcare when you have your new baby.

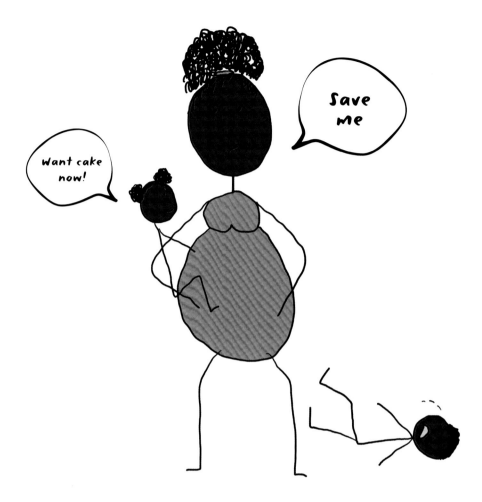

/ PREPARE YOUR LITTLE ONE FOR THE NEW ARRIVAL

You could get a book about being a big brother or sister, or even help them to create a painting/picture for them to give to the baby – this helps with feelings of inclusion. Talk to your toddler about the things that might change when the baby arrives, i.e. sharing cuddles, and show them where the nappies will be so they can fetch them to lend a hand. If they are big enough, get them to start climbing into their car seat rather than you lifting them, and practise being independent, i.e. putting on clothes and washing themselves. You may feel like it's a lot to ask of them being so young, but it's a good place to start. It also helps them develop a sense of independence!

Encourage your toddler to bond with the baby by singing or speaking to your belly and asking them what names they like. Ask them if they want to feel the baby moving and listen to the heartbeat at your midwife appointments.

Breastfeeding While Pregnant

Breastfeeding your baby or toddler while pregnant is absolutely fine in the majority of cases. Some people worry about their milk supply dwindling, and become concerned that if they feed a toddler, there won't be anything left for baby when they are born, or that it will kickstart a premature labour.

I'm going to break down common concerns regarding breastfeeding while pregnant:

- Your body will usually continue making milk while you're pregnant, so you'll be able to breastfeed. Some women, however, notice a reduction in their milk supply due to the hormonal changes that occur.

- You may feel some cramps low down in your womb when feeding, which is caused by the oxytocin hormone being triggered by the action of breastfeeding. They shouldn't be strong enough to send you into labour or cause a miscarriage, however if you are considered a high risk for miscarriage or preterm labour, you might want to discuss this with your midwife or doctor first.

- When your baby is born, your milk should change to suit your newborn. You may even find at this point that your toddler doesn't want to feed as much as they previously did.

Some toddlers will wean themselves off the breast due to the change in milk and you may even find that hormonal changes cause it to dry up during pregnancy. When the new baby is born however, the milk supply will naturally increase again. Many women go on to feed both a baby and a toddler in tandem; it's totally your call!

Fibroids

Intramural fibroids

Submucosal fibroids

Uterus

Many people with fibroids, particularly small ones, have no problems. Occasionally though, fibroids can cause complications with the development and birth of the baby, depending on their size and location.

The uterine fibroid, also known as leiomyoma or myoma, is a mass of compacted muscle and fibrous tissue that sometimes grows on the wall (or sometimes on the outside) of the uterus. Fibroids can be small like a pea, or as large as a grapefruit. They usually occur before pregnancy but most women won't know they have them until they have had an ultrasound. Fibroids are actually quite common; you may know someone who has them!

One complication associated with fibroids is excess bleeding after birth (postpartum haemorrhage) if the uterus struggles to contract back down because the fibroids are in the way. Depending on the location and size, some fibroids may obstruct the birth canal, making a vaginal birth difficult. If a fibroid is detected on ultrasound, the sonographer will document the size and report back to the midwife or obstetrician. They will then discuss the plan of care with you and monitor you accordingly.

Some people have a higher risk of developing fibroids than others. Risk factors for uterine fibroids include:

- **Age** – They are more common in older mothers.
- **Ethnicity** – They are more common in black women.
- **Family history** – If a close female relative has had fibroids.
- **High blood pressure.**

Fibroids don't make labour contractions more uncomfortable, but some women who are known to have large ones may choose to have them surgically removed prior to conceiving. As well as potentially reducing pregnancy and birth-related complications, removal of fibroids can help reduce abdominal pain and heavy periods when not pregnant.

Common Pregnancy Complaints

Some pregnancies are plain sailing, while others are met with lots of niggles, the majority of which are thankfully not serious. This section covers some of the most frequent pregnancy complaints.

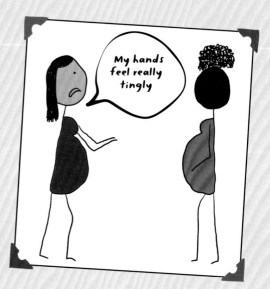

Carpal tunnel syndrome

Carpal tunnel syndrome is a fairly common condition that can sometimes occur during pregnancy.

The carpal tunnel is a narrow passage in the wrist, made up of small bones and a strong band of tissue. Within the tunnel are tendons, blood vessels and nerves including the median nerve, which controls sensation and movement in the hand. Compression of this nerve is defined as carpal tunnel syndrome and it can cause a range of strange sensations, including tingling and numbness in your fingers.

If your hands become swollen (oedematous) during pregnancy, some of the fluid can collect in the carpal tunnel, putting pressure on the median nerve.

Around 60 per cent of people experience symptoms of carpal tunnel syndrome during pregnancy. They can range in severity, usually being worse first thing in the morning and at night.

Aside from numbness and tingling, symptoms which could signal carpal tunnel syndrome include:

- Pain or throbbing in the fingers, wrists or forearm.
- Swollen, hot fingers and thumb.
- Difficulty gripping objects.

If you are suffering from carpal tunnel syndrome, there are some things you can do to help reduce severity of symptoms.

Try to avoid over-using your hands where possible. For example, if you spend a lot of time texting, experiment with using the 'speak to text' option on your phone instead. If you use a computer a lot at work, talk to your employer about other activities you may be able to do, or reducing the workload, to avoid typing too much.

Applying an icepack for five to ten minutes or holding your hand under a cold running tap may help alleviate discomfort and swelling.

Although resting your hands is important, doing specific hand/wrist exercises is also a good way of relieving pressure on the median nerve.

Try the following daily:

- Keeping your fingers straight, bend your wrist forwards and backwards. Repeat this ten times.
- Make a fist, then open and straighten your fingers. Repeat this ten times.
- Touch each finger one at a time with the thumb of your same hand, making an 'o' shape.

If symptoms become extreme, seek advice from your GP who may refer you to a physiotherapist.

Carpal tunnel syndrome thankfully usually disappears after pregnancy.

Haemorrhoids

Haemorrhoids, also known as piles, are swellings containing enlarged blood vessels inside or around the rectum and anus. You can get them at any time, but they are pretty common in pregnancy because the change in hormones makes your veins relax. If you've managed to escape them in pregnancy, you may end up getting them postnatally as a result of pushing your baby out. Or you may just be lucky and not get them at all!

Symptoms of piles can include:

- Itching, aching, soreness or swelling around your anus.
- Pain when pooping and a mucus discharge afterwards.
- A lump hanging outside the anus.
- Bleeding after pooping – the blood is usually bright red.

Constipation can cause haemorrhoids, so be sure to include plenty of fibre in your diet and drink lots of water.

Tips to help relieve the discomfort:

- Hold a cold, wet cloth against the area to soothe it.
- If the piles stick out, push them gently back inside using a lubricating jelly.
- Avoid straining when you go to the toilet, as this may make them worse.
- After going to the toilet, clean yourself with moist instead of dry toilet paper, and pat the area dry rather than rubbing it.

Some medicines can help soothe inflammation around your anus. These treat the symptoms, but not the cause, of piles. Ask your pharmacist or doctor for medication that might help, if necessary.

Headaches

Hormonal changes mean headaches may happen quite a bit in the first few months but tend to get better by the time you're around 6 months' pregnant. Keeping yourself hydrated, ensuring you get enough sleep, and avoiding stress, can all help reduce headaches.

Sometimes headaches after 20 weeks of pregnancy can be a sign of pre-eclampsia, which can cause complications if it's not monitored and treated.

If you experience any of the following symptoms along with your headache, contact your doctor/midwife/hospital straight away:

- A sudden severe headache, or one that is getting progressively worse.
- Chest pain or pain just below the ribs on the right.
- Visual disturbances/flashing lights/ seeing spots.
- Vomiting.
- Sudden severe swelling to your face, hands, legs/feet.

The vast majority of headaches in pregnancy are absolutely harmless, but it's always worthwhile making a note of unusual symptoms and contacting your care provider for further advice. Paracetamol is safe to take in pregnancy for headaches and most headaches, you'll be glad to know, are short lived.

Backache

As pregnancy progresses, several changes occur in the body that can contribute to backache: the joints of the pelvis start to soften and the growing uterus can throw you a little off-balance. To compensate for this, you may find that you inadvertently throw your hips forward and shoulders back. As a result, the lower back becomes more curved and the back muscles are strained, sometimes causing pain.

To help prevent backache, make sure you sit correctly (avoid slouching and sit up straight with feet flat on the floor or on a footstool) and avoid sitting for long periods of time (sitting down puts extra pressure on the back). Using a footstool to raise your knees so that they are in line with your hips, and sitting in a chair that reclines slightly, can both help to take the pressure off. If you sit for long periods of time at work, speak to your employer when they conduct the risk assessment to see if they can provide you with an orthopaedic chair and footstool. Standing for long periods can also cause pain and discomfort: if you have to stand to work, try putting one foot on a stool to relieve some of the pressure on your back.

Take care when lifting things. Avoid lifting heavy loads where possible, but if you have to lift, do it slowly, bending at the knees rather than at the hips while picking up items. If you have to carry multiple items, spread the load evenly in both arms. You may even want to consider an abdominal support belt to take some of the pressure of your bump off your back. Wear comfortable low-heeled shoes as much as possible.

If you have other children, you might be wondering whether it's okay to lift them. Lifting your toddler for short periods while pregnant is not thought to cause any harm, unless your care provider has advised you otherwise.

Sciatic nerve pain

Some people suffer from sciatic nerve pain in pregnancy. Personally, pregnancy was the only time when I've ever suffered from it! I remember clearly, at 14 weeks' pregnant, when all of a sudden I had this shooting pain from my bum down my leg. It was made worse when I walked.

The sciatic nerve is a huge nerve that runs down your leg from your lower back. Pain may come in the form of a dull ache, or a shooting or stabbing feeling. Some women even complain of a tingling or burning-type pain. Lumbar spine problems such as a herniated disc are often a cause of sciatica but, during pregnancy, sciatic pain can often have other causes. Sciatic-like symptoms are common with lower back pain and also may be caused by unstable joints and even muscle tension.

Sciatica is not caused by pregnancy but if you do happen to suffer from it when pregnant it could be related to increased weight and fluid retention putting pressure on the nerve or even your centre of gravity being pushed forward, meaning you subconsciously clench your buttocks more, pinching the sciatic nerve! Certain stretches, yoga positions and massage can help relieve discomfort.

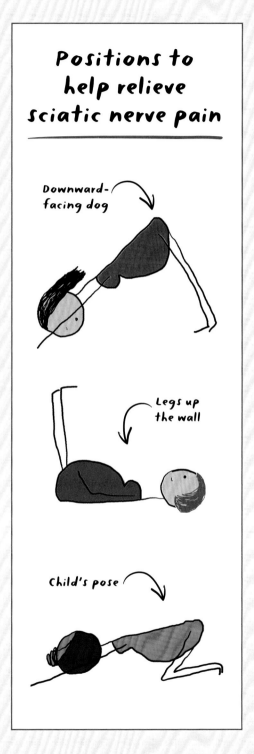

Positions to help relieve sciatic nerve pain

Downward-facing dog

Legs up the wall

Child's pose

Heart palpitations

Your body carries extra blood when you're pregnant and this can cause your heart rate to increase so it beats about 25 per cent faster than usual. A faster heart rate can result in occasional heart palpitations which feel like your heart is racing, thumping or even skipping a beat (ectopic beats). Stress and anxiety can exacerbate the symptoms too.

In the vast majority of cases, heart palpitations in pregnancy are no cause for concern, but in rare situations it can be caused by pre-eclampsia, hypertension, underlying heart disorders or thyroid problems.

Always mention heart palpitations to your care provider. If you are also experiencing chest pain or shortness of breath, seek medical attention straight away. There are simple investigations that can be done to rule out any serious causes of palpitations.

Round ligament pain

The uterus (womb) grows rapidly throughout pregnancy, which in turn can cause discomfort known as round ligament pain. The uterus only measures around 7–8cm pre-pregnancy, growing to about 40cm when you are ready to give birth at around 40 weeks. That's a lot of growing!

The uterus needs to be held in position, otherwise it would flop all over the place, so it has a couple of ligaments either side that keep it steady.

As the uterus grows, the ligaments also stretch and thin, which can cause a sharp stabbing sensation, or even a dull ache in your groin. Usually, it only happens on one side or another, but occasionally it can occur on both sides. You may feel pain briefly for a few seconds, or it may repeat on and off throughout the day, but it should not be there constantly. The pain might be triggered if you move quickly, sneeze or cough forcefully. Round ligament pain won't harm the baby, but it is pretty annoying and uncomfortable for you!

When I ran my antenatal clinic, almost every person who attended their 16-week appointment would mention this pain. It can occur at any time during pregnancy but is more common at 13–17 weeks, a time when the uterus has risen out of the pelvis and the ligaments are starting to feel the strain.

You can help to reduce discomfort by wearing a belly support band, going easy with exercise and moving out of chairs/ changing positions slowly.

As with ANY abdominal pain you experience in pregnancy, if it becomes severe, constant, or is accompanied by vaginal bleeding, be sure to seek advice from your care provider.

Swelling (oedema)

A slight swelling in feet, ankles and hands is a frequent complaint in pregnancy and is usually due to the excess fluid that is held in your body and the increase in blood volume.

Swelling can be pretty uncomfortable, especially at the end of the day or if you have been standing for too long! You may find that shoes, watches and rings become too tight, and that this is often exacerbated by walking a lot. Around 75 per cent of people will suffer from swelling at some point during pregnancy, and it is likely to be more noticeable in hot weather or at the end of the day.

Avoiding long periods of sitting or standing may help, as may keeping your legs elevated when you are resting. Don't reduce your fluid intake in the hope that the swelling will reduce. It will most likely make it worse if you are dehydrated.

Swelling may continue for a little while after the birth, especially if you have IV (intravenous) fluids during labour or caesarean. Swelling can sometimes, however, be an indication of a problem. A sudden, extreme case of swelling that occurs after 20 weeks of pregnancy can be a sign of pre-eclampsia. For this reason, any incidence of swelling should be mentioned to your care provider.

Discharge

Vaginal discharge is normal whether you're pregnant or not. During pregnancy, however, you may notice that the amount and consistency of discharge changes. Thin, white, odourless, milky discharge, known as leucorrhoea, is fine. It may be more noticeable at the beginning of pregnancy and then again towards the end. This discharge helps protect the birth canal from infection and keep the vaginal flora (colonies of healthy bacteria) balanced and healthy. If the discharge becomes heavy, you may want to wear panty liners to make you feel more comfortable.

If you notice any vaginal discharge that smells unusual, or is abnormally coloured, i.e. green/grey, or are suffering from vaginal irritation such as burning or itching, this may be indicative of an infection. You should always mention this to your care provider.

Shortness of breath

Lots of women experience some mild shortness of breath at certain points throughout their pregnancy and it's usually harmless, but there are times when shortness of breath can indicate a more serious problem.

Why does shortness of breath occur? During early pregnancy, the increase in the progesterone hormone can cause you to breathe more often, giving you a feeling of being short of breath (the hormone expands your lung capacity, allowing you to carry more oxygen to the baby). Low iron levels are also associated with feeling short of breath.

As your pregnancy progresses, the uterus starts to squash other organs, and your diaphragm, which makes it harder for your lungs to fully expand.

If you have gained a lot of weight rapidly, or don't exercise regularly, you may also be more likely to feel short of breath. This doesn't mean those who kept active before pregnancy are exempt, however! So, when should you be concerned? Shortness of breath should always be mentioned to your care provider regardless of other symptoms, but seek advice without delay if:

- You have other symptoms such as chest pain, arm pain, vomiting, headaches, dizziness, palpitations or visual disturbances (e.g. flashing lights, floaters/seeing spots, blurred vision).
- You have a history of pulmonary embolism (PE) or heart problems.
- The shortness of breath onset is very sudden, is severe, and is restricting you from doing the slightest things, such as walking to the other side of the room.
- You are feeling unwell, confused, or have a sense of 'impending doom'.
- You have a cough that doesn't go away, or coughing up blood.
- You notice blueness around the lips, fingers or toes. You may not notice lip-colour changes in people with dark skin – it may be detected through the fingernails and mucous membranes such as the mouth instead.

Restless leg syndrome

Restless leg syndrome (RLS) in pregnancy is a thing! RLS affects about one in five people during pregnancy and can be particularly aggravating and uncomfortable. The need to move your legs is caused by crawling, creeping or tingling sensations. You may have these feelings inside your foot, calf or upper leg. Sometimes you'll feel aching, cramping or a fidgety feeling, but above all you'll have an overpowering urge to move your legs. It's usually worse at night, and can be a real pain in the neck when you're trying to wind down and sleep.

RLS usually occurs in the third trimester and there isn't much you can do to get rid of it for good, although reducing caffeine intake, taking exercise, and giving your leg a massage can bring temporary relief.

It is thought that RLS could be linked to iron deficiency in pregnancy. Some doctors suggest magnesium supplements may help, but discuss this with your care provider before you start taking any supplements.

Varicose veins

You may have noticed large, non-painful, swollen-looking veins popping out in your legs. These are probably varicose veins. Varicose veins aren't limited to the legs however: they may show up in the vulva or even around your rectum – haemorrhoids (see page 53) are quite simply varicose veins that are around your bum! Many get varicose veins confused with spider veins.

Spider veins are very thin purplish-looking vessels that sit flat under the skin.

Varicose veins swell above the surface of the skin and affect up to 40 per cent of women during pregnancy. Varicose veins are often genetic, so if there is a strong family history of them, it's more likely you will get them too. They can become more pronounced in pregnancy due to the extra pressure put on the vessels while they're working hard to push the extra blood back up to the heart.

Varicose veins will usually reduce in size, and may even disappear completely, once you have had your baby.

If you suffer from varicose veins, or want to help prevent them, here are some tips that may help:

- Keep moving – Don't spend long periods on your feet, and keep legs elevated when sitting. Try to avoid sitting with your legs crossed.
- Exercise – This is key when it comes to preventing varicose veins. Taking a walk or two each day will help keep the blood flowing around your body, preventing pressure building up. Swimming is also a great exercise to help promote a healthy circulatory system.
- Wear comfortable clothes that fit well. Avoid clothes that are tight in areas such as your ankles and thighs.
- Eat healthily to avoid excessive weight gain, as too much weight can put pressure on your circulatory system.

If you develop a painful swelling in your leg (which can appear red in people with fair skin), seek advice without delay from your care provider as it may be a sign of a deep vein thrombosis (DVT).

This is ultimately a blood clot that develops in your leg and would require immediate attention.

Leg cramps

Leg cramps are pretty painful at any time, but during pregnancy they seem to be ten times worse and happen more often, especially at night! Leg cramps are simply the muscle contracting – usually the calf muscle – and not relaxing. Sometimes you can even see the muscle change shape! No one really knows for sure why leg cramps happen more often in pregnancy, but some theories include lack of calcium or magnesium and fatigue/dehydration.

If you have leg cramps, try flexing your foot up and down vigorously and, if that doesn't work, pull your toes up towards your ankle until the feeling subsides. If you can't manage it yourself, get your partner to help you. Sometimes a good foot massage helps, too.

Doing stretching exercises before bed may help prevent leg cramps at night. Around 30-60 minutes before you get into bed, try stretching your calves by leaning on a wall with your hands, with your feet around 50cm from the wall. As you lean forward, keep your heels flat on the ground and you should feel the stretch in the thighs and calves. Magnesium or calcium supplements may help, but speak to your care provider before taking either of these.

I had terrible leg cramps when I was pregnant with my youngest child, to the point where I leapt out of bed in the middle of the night to stretch my feet on the wall! You'll be glad to know, leg cramps almost always disappear after pregnancy.

Lightning crotch

It's a bit of a dramatic name, but 'lightning crotch' is a good way to describe the shooting pain that some people complain of in the groin during pregnancy. Once in a while, you may feel a very sudden and intense 'electric shock' or stabbing-type pain that feels like it's deep within your groin or vagina. The sensation can be so intense that it takes your breath away for a few seconds, and can last for several minutes before subsiding, and it can happen even when you are sitting down and haven't exerted yourself in any way.

This phenomenon has no real explanation or even a medical name, but it's quite common in the second and third trimesters. Some theories suggest it could be to do with the baby pressing on a nerve that runs to the cervix as they shuffle around in the uterus.

Pelvic girdle pain

Pelvic girdle pain (PGP), sometimes called symphysis pubis dysfunction, refers to an array of uncomfortable symptoms in the pelvic area, caused by joint instability or stiffness. This can occur at either the back or front of your pelvis. Symptoms of PGP include pain over the pubic bone at the front, which can feel tender to touch and may hurt when moving, and you might also experience pain across your lower back, perineum, and/or thighs. Movements that require leg opening, such as walking, getting out of bed or walking up the stairs, may make the pain worse. If you suffer from PGP, take your time with these movements and try to keep your legs together when rolling over and getting out of bed. If you feel that the discomfort is having a severe impact on you and your ability to function normally throughout the day, seek advice from your GP who may be able to refer you to a physiotherapist.

PGP is not harmful to your baby, but it may make moving around difficult for you. Some people suffer more than others, but PGP alone should not affect your ability to have a vaginal birth.

Constipation

That feeling of being clogged up, windy and unable to pass stools regularly is a very common pregnancy complaint. High levels of the hormone progesterone during pregnancy cause the smooth muscles in the bowel to relax, making them sluggish.

Many people who are pregnant don't drink enough water, which also contributes to constipation, as does the uterus putting pressure on the bowels, inhibiting its usual activity. You may notice constipation more at the beginning of pregnancy and in the third trimester. Constipation can be miserable; chronic episodes can cause abdominal pain and uncomfortable haemorrhoids from excessive straining on the toilet.

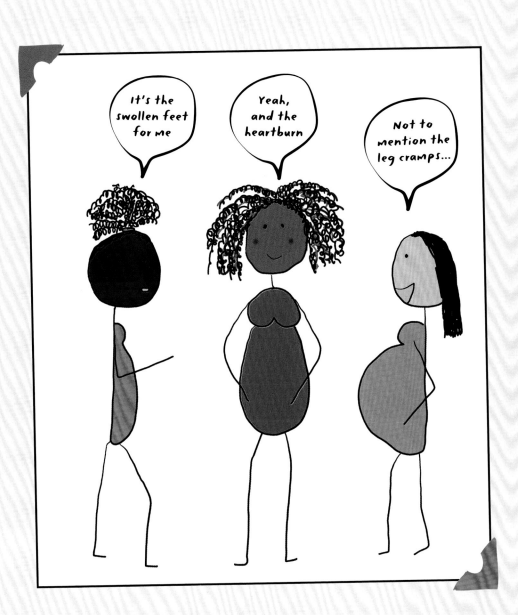

Eating more fibrous foods such as wholemeal breads and cereals, pulses and greens, along with increasing fluid intake, can help. Some iron supplements can cause constipation. If you have low iron levels and have been prescribed them, speak to your doctor about changing to a different type.

Heartburn

Heartburn, also called acid reflux or indigestion, is common in pregnancy. A combination of your growing uterus pressing on the stomach, and hormonal changes, can cause the valve at the entrance to the stomach to relax so that it doesn't close as it should. This in turn allows acid from the stomach to travel up the oesophagus, which can be felt as a burning sensation or pain in the chest area. You may also belch a lot, feel nauseous or vomit, have a feeling of fullness, or notice small lumps of food regurgitating into your mouth. These symptoms commonly occur shortly after eating.

Changing your eating and drinking habits may help improve heartburn. Eating several small meals per day rather than fewer large ones, and avoiding eating too close to bedtime (within three hours of going to bed), are steps you can take. Try to steer clear of very spicy foods and carbonated drinks, too.

If you are struggling to manage symptoms, unable to keep food or drink down, losing weight, or experiencing abdominal pain, speak with your midwife or doctor.

There is an old wives' tale that if a woman has heartburn during pregnancy, the baby will be born with lots of hair. It's considered a myth, but there may actually be some science behind it.

In 2006, US researchers at Johns Hopkins Hospital in Baltimore, USA, carried out a study with 64 pregnant women. They concluded that women who had suffered moderate heartburn had newborns with more hair, 82 per cent of the time. The majority of heartburn-free women gave birth to bald babies. Their theory for why this happened is down to hormones again. This was quite a small study, so much more needs to be done before the link between heartburn and babies with lots of hair can be said to be conclusive.

My first son was born with thick black hair that was over 5cm long. He was the only child I had where I suffered severe heartburn, so who knows – perhaps there is something to be said about the old wives' tale!

Complications In Pregnancy

Developing a complication during pregnancy is something that many people worry about. It doesn't help when you read about negative birth stories, or worse, someone tells you about theirs while you are pregnant! Although, thankfully, the majority of pregnancies are straightforward without complications, there are occasions when an issue is detected.

This is why antenatal care is so important, as is being in tune with your body and understanding when to reach out if something doesn't feel right.

Pre-eclampsia

Pre-eclampsia, which can occur in the second half of pregnancy, is a condition thought to be caused by a placenta that hasn't developed properly, and issues with the blood vessels within it, however the exact cause is not fully understood. It is characterised by high blood pressure, protein in the urine and sudden swelling in the body. In most cases, it is resolved with the birth of the baby. Occasionally though, pre-eclampsia can develop after the pregnancy, and then it is known as postpartum pre-eclampsia. This can lead to serious complications such as HELLP syndrome (a rare condition that affects your liver and blood). If pre-eclampsia is left untreated, it can become severe, turning into eclampsia which can cause seizures, organ failure and even death.

Initially, pre-eclampsia may present no symptoms, however early signs include:

- High blood pressure (hypertension).
- Protein in the urine (proteinuria).

In most cases, a woman will not be aware of these two signs until a midwife observes her during an antenatal visit.

As the pre-eclampsia progresses, the woman may experience fluid retention (oedema), with swelling in the hands, feet, ankles and face.

Swelling is common in pregnancy, especially during the third trimester, and tends to occur in the ankles and feet. Symptoms are typically milder first thing in the morning and build up during the day. In pre-eclampsia, it's different; oedema occurs suddenly and tends to be much more severe.

The following signs and symptoms may also develop:

- Blurry vision, sometimes seeing flashing lights.
- Severe headache.
- Feeling generally unwell.
- Shortness of breath.

- Pain just below the ribs on the right side.
- Rapid weight gain (caused by fluid retention).
- Vomiting.

If you experience sudden onset of any of these symptoms, be sure to mention it to your care provider even if you have recently given birth.

Gestational diabetes

Gestational diabetes occurs when you have high levels of glucose in your blood during pregnancy. It usually develops in the third trimester (after 28 weeks) and disappears after the baby is born. Women who develop gestational diabetes are more likely to develop Type 2 diabetes later on in life.

The hormonal changes in the second and third trimesters of pregnancy, along with the growth demands of the foetus, increase a pregnant woman's insulin needs by two to three times that of normal. Insulin takes the sugar from your blood and moves it into your body's cells for energy. If your body cannot make this amount of insulin, sugar from the foods you eat will stay in your bloodstream and cause high blood sugars. This is gestational diabetes. It occurs in around one in twenty pregnancies and is usually detected through routine blood sugar or urine tests when you visit your doctor or midwife in pregnancy.

If you are told you have gestational diabetes, a specialist midwife and obstetrician will work with you to ensure your blood sugar levels remain stable, usually via dietary changes and/or medication. You will also be advised to keep a record of your blood sugar levels at home with the use of a finger-prick device. Without these measures, people with gestational diabetes would be more likely to suffer from complications.

Some factors which increase the risk of developing gestational diabetes include:

- Age over 35.
- Family history of diabetes.
- Obesity.
- People who have Black, South Asian and Middle Eastern backgrounds.

If you have any of the risk factors above, you may be offered a special test around 26-28 weeks to assess your tolerance to glucose.

Obstetric cholestasis

Obstetric cholestasis is a liver disorder. In the unlikely event that it is suspected, your midwife or doctor will order a blood test to see how well your liver is working and will also measure your bile acids.

Most women diagnosed with obstetric cholestasis will go on to have healthy babies following close monitoring and regular blood tests; in some cases an earlier birth may be recommended.

Pregnancy-induced hypertension

If you are pregnant and have a history of high blood pressure (hypertension), or have developed high blood pressure for the first time in pregnancy, you will be monitored carefully by your care provider. According to the NHS, high blood pressure in pregnancy falls into three categories:

- **Mild** – Blood pressure between 140/90 and 149/99mmHg (millimetres of mercury); the person may be checked regularly but does not usually need treatment.
- **Moderate** – Blood pressure between 150/100 and 159/109mmHg.
- **Severe** – Blood pressure of 160/110mmHg or higher.

If you already take medication for hypertension and find out you're pregnant, inform your doctor as soon as possible, as they may need to change your medication to one that is safe for use in pregnancy. Some women suffer from hypertension that occurs in pregnancy and disappears a while after. It still needs to be monitored, and treated if it gets too high.

Other women may develop hypertension after 20 weeks due to pre-eclampsia (see pages 63-64). If your blood pressure appears to be within the normal range, but it has risen significantly from when you had your first antenatal appointment and other symptoms are present too, it may be a reason for your care provider to investigate further.

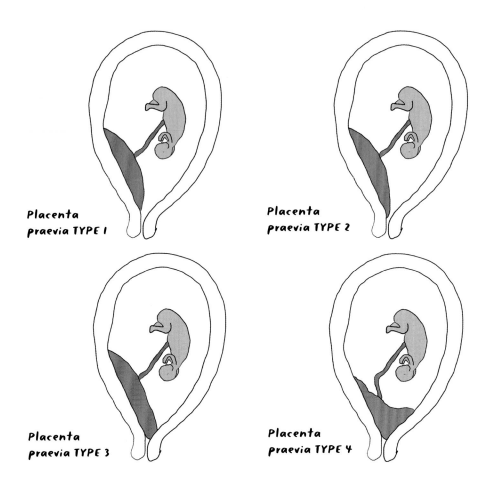

Placenta praevia TYPE 1

Placenta praevia TYPE 2

Placenta praevia TYPE 3

Placenta praevia TYPE 4

Antenatal haemorrhage

Antenatal haemorrhage (APH) is bleeding from the vagina that can occur after 24 weeks of pregnancy. This is different to spotting where there are a few spots of pink or brown blood on wiping. APH often requires a pad to be worn and the bleeding can sometimes soak through several. Around 20 per cent of preterm babies are born as a result of APH. In more concerning cases, it is caused by an issue with the placenta:

/ **PLACENTA PRAEVIA**. When the placenta is growing too close to the cervix, potentially blocking the baby from being born. There are different types of placenta praevia as illustrated above. (A complete placenta praevia will always necessitate a caesarean birth and will often result in vaginal bleeding throughout pregnancy.)

/ **PLACENTAL ABRUPTION**. When the placenta has started to separate from the lining of the uterus. The way this is managed will depend on how well mother and baby are, along with the nature of the abruption. Close monitoring or an emergency caesarean may be necessary.

Other causes of bleeding can include infection or cervical ectropion (when cells from inside the cervical canal are present on the outside surface of the cervix). You may find that you bleed a little after sexual intercourse if the cervix is irritated. Any type of bleeding in pregnancy should always be mentioned to your care provider.

IUGR (intrauterine growth restriction)

IUGR is the term used when a baby is not growing as they should be in the womb. Sometimes the phrase 'small for gestational age' is used interchangeably with IUGR, but it has a different meaning. 'Small for gestational age' doesn't necessarily mean the baby is growth restricted, it simply means the baby appears to be much smaller than average. This could be normal for a baby whose parents are both smaller than the general population.

To determine if a baby is actually growth restricted by other factors, tests will need to be performed and medical history reviewed. If your care provider suspects baby isn't growing well, you will be given a growth ultrasound scan. This scan can also provide information on how the placenta is functioning. IUGR can be caused by a number of factors, including:

- Maternal weight less than 43kg/ extremely low or high BMI.
- Poor nutrition during pregnancy.
- Birth defects or chromosomal abnormalities.
- Drug-taking.
- Smoking.

- Heavy alcohol use.
- High blood pressure.
- Placental abnormalities.
- Umbilical cord abnormalities.
- Twins/triplets or more.
- Gestational diabetes.
- Low levels of amniotic fluid.

It is estimated that 3–7 per cent of unborn babies have IUGR and one of the noticeable signs that some mothers experience is reduced foetal movements. This is especially true if there is an issue with the placenta. The plan of care depends on your gestation at the time of discovering IUGR, and the severity. Some babies are monitored closely and are born at full term, others are induced a little early, particularly if it's found that the placenta is not working as it should.

Although it may be daunting to think about issues arising during pregnancy, it's good to remember that in the unlikely event of a problem, your care provider will work with you to ensure the best health of both you and your baby.

Foetal Movements

'When will I feel my baby move?!' This is one of the questions I'm most frequently asked.

We all want to feel those first flutters because a) it's reassuring to feel that there really is a baby in there, and b) it helps us to bond with our baby during pregnancy. For many women who have previously suffered an early miscarriage, the first movements are an extremely important marker.

When you feel the first flutters of movement varies from woman to woman. The range of when you may feel movements is vast – typically anywhere between 13 and 23 weeks. The baby generally has to be big enough to be able to move so that they touch your uterus in order for you to be able to feel it. If you have had a baby before, you will know what to look out for and will probably feel the baby moving earlier than you did first time around. If it's your first, however, it's more common to start feeling the baby move after 18 weeks. You may be aware of a flutter, wonder if it's the baby, and then not notice anything again for a few more days. The first movement may feel like bubbles, flutters, or even a twitch!

As your baby gets bigger, the movements become stronger and you can start to feel more defined kicks, nudges and twists. You should notice your baby developing a more regular pattern of movement too; generally speaking there will be some sort of daily rhythm by the time you are around 26–28 weeks' pregnant.

Sometimes the position of the placenta may affect when you first feel foetal movements. If your placenta is in an anterior position, it can act as a cushion for movements at the front of the uterus, so you may not feel them until a little later. Regardless of the position of the placenta however, if you haven't felt any movements by 24 weeks, reach out to your care provider for advice.

Any episode of reduced or stopping of movement warrants a call to your care provider without delay. Never ignore reduced baby movements; never feel that you are 'bothering' your care provider. Always trust your instincts and don't sleep on it to see if baby 'wakes up a bit' in the morning.

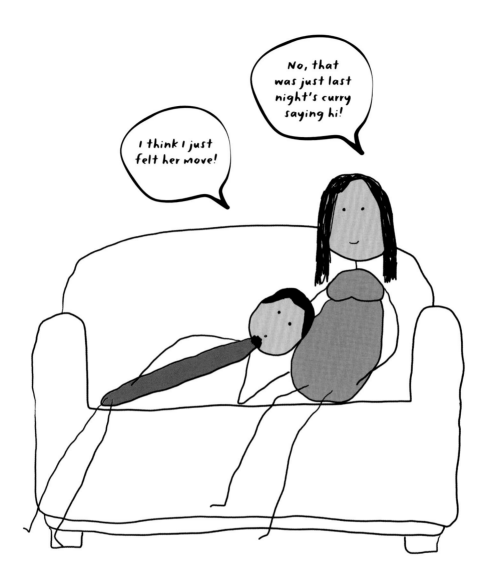

Is it true that later in pregnancy babies move less?

You may hear that babies move less at the end of pregnancy. There is no truth in this. Yes, their movements may change from sharp kicks to sliding and rolling movements which might not feel as intense, but the frequency of these movements should still remain the same.

Braxton Hicks Contractions

Braxton Hicks contractions are basically practice contractions that don't result in the birth of a baby. It's the process of the uterus tightening and relaxing several times per day to prepare for the big day!

Braxton Hicks contractions occur throughout pregnancy, but most women don't feel them until around 20 weeks and some don't notice them at all! Some women, including me, will feel them much earlier than 20 weeks, especially if they have had children before.

Braxton Hicks contractions aren't usually painful, but they can feel strange and uncomfortable, and change the shape of your abdomen momentarily.

Braxton Hicks contractions tend to increase in intensity towards the end of pregnancy and some women report that occasionally the contractions have taken their breath away! If you are full term and have these tightenings that gradually become more painful and frequent over time like a worsening period cramp, it could be that the Braxton Hicks are transitioning into real labour contractions. It doesn't always mean that though – you can have prolonged periods of frequent Braxton Hicks contractions and then they just disappear.

As a general rule, if you are pre 37 weeks and are experiencing five or more of these tightenings per hour, call your care provider. We want to avoid them turning into real labour contractions if you are preterm. Sometimes, Braxton Hicks contractions can increase in intensity and volume if you are dehydrated, so it's important to make sure you drink plenty of water throughout pregnancy.

You may also find that you experience really intense Braxton Hicks contractions after intercourse or orgasm!

Foetal Positions

There are several positions that a baby may get themselves into ready for the birth, and the position can have an impact on the birth process itself. By 36 weeks, most babies manage to get themselves into a head-down position. Being head down is what we want and expect a baby to be.

There are two main types of head-down (cephalic) position however – occiput anterior (OA) and occiput posterior (OP), which are illustrated below. The occiput is the name given to the back of the head. The optimal position for your baby to be in is OA: the head is down, the face is looking towards your spine and their back is resting against your belly. This means that they can exit the birth canal with the back of their head closest to your pubic bone, making it easier for them to rotate through the pelvis.

Sometimes a baby may not be lying in this optimal position during labour, which can make labour more challenging.

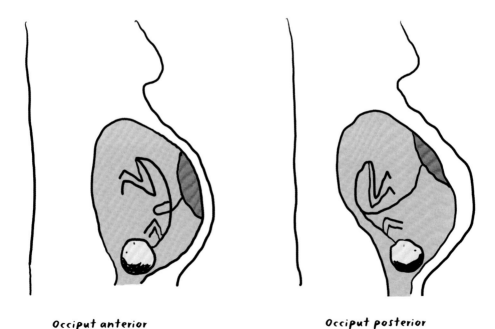

Occiput anterior

Occiput posterior

An example of this is a baby that is lying in the OP position. The baby is head down, but instead of the baby facing your spine, they are looking at your belly with their back running along your spine. This is also known as 'back to back' or 'sunny-side up'. In this position, the baby can't flex their head down properly as they are making their way through the birth canal, and as a result labour can take longer. Some babies are born this way vaginally, and others may be born via caesarean if the baby is finding it a struggle to come down.

Other unusual positions include breech – baby is bum, knee or feet first as opposed to head – transverse (the baby is lying horizontally across the abdomen), and oblique (the baby is lying diagonally).

A breech baby may be born vaginally with the help of an experienced doctor or midwife, or a caesarean may be offered. A transverse or oblique baby that won't turn (so that either the bum or head is in the pelvis) will need to be born via caesarean. Sometimes, though, babies get into a good position at the last minute so your doctor and/or midwife will monitor the situation.

Getting your baby into a good position

To help get baby into an optimal position, regularly use upright and forward leaning positions. This will encourage more pelvic space for the baby. You can also try the following:

- When you sit, aim to have your knees lower than your hips, with your back as straight as possible. When reading, try sitting at a table, with your arms on the table, knees apart, torso leaning slightly forward.

- Kneel on the floor with your body draped over a bean bag or cushion. You can do this while watching television.

- When resting, lie on your left side with a pillow between your legs, with the higher knee extended over so it's resting on the bed.

- Try 'child's pose', a yoga position which you can see illustrated on page 55.

- The 'Miles Circuit' illustrates a few positions that can also help optimise the baby's position in pregnancy and during labour. It can be found at *milescircuit.com*

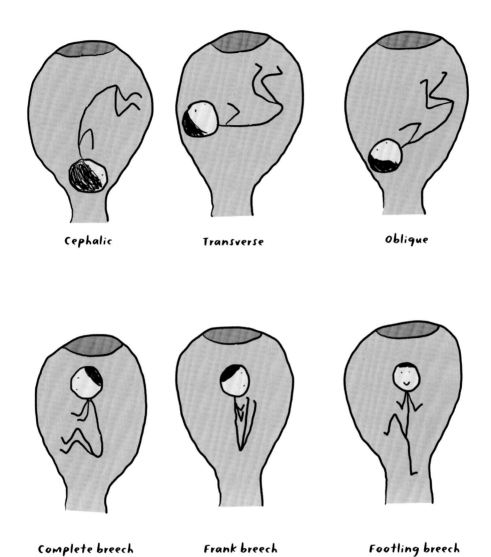

Cephalic   Transverse   Oblique

Complete breech   Frank breech   Footling breech

Twins And Multiples

So, you went for an ultrasound only to be told you are growing more than one baby. It's a complete shock, right?

In 2007 I was told I was going to have two babies – I totally understand how daunting it is. Expecting twins, triplets or more is a pretty formidable prospect and you will no doubt be feeling a range of emotions and thoughts, varying from 'this is totally amazing' to 'how on earth am I/are we going to cope?'.

You won't know if you are pregnant with more than one baby until you have an ultrasound scan, but it could be more likely if you have had assisted conception such as IVF, or if you have pregnancy symptoms such as nausea extremely early.

Twins and multiples can be more complex than singleton pregnancies, so it is likely you will be offered care from an obstetric doctor, often in conjunction with a midwife. Twins and multiples need additional monitoring during pregnancy, so you may find you have extra ultrasound scans and more appointments with the doctor.

The plan of care for the birth will vary greatly from pregnancy to pregnancy and will depend on factors such as whether or not the babies share a placenta and/or membranes (the sacs around them), the position and wellbeing of the babies, and if there are any maternal medical issues. Contrary to popular belief, twins aren't always born by caesarean. Many people have successful vaginal births.

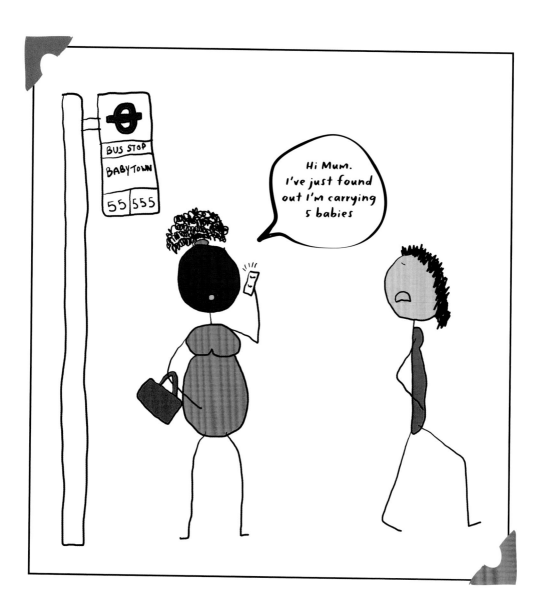

Work And Maternity Leave

Employers have responsibilities when it comes to the wellbeing of their pregnant employees while they're still at work.

You may be wondering how your work will be affected when you have a baby, but you'll be glad to hear that in the UK you are legally entitled to 52 weeks' leave as an employee. This means that your job has to remain open to you when this time is up, and you can begin your leave any time from the 28th week of pregnancy.

In the UK it is compulsory for you to take at least 2 weeks' leave after giving birth, or 4 weeks if you work in a factory. It takes time to heal after having a baby, so the more time you have off the better. It also supports bonding with your baby. Pay wise, each employer may have a different scheme, but statutory maternity pay (SMP) is available for eligible employees. The first 6 weeks is 90 per cent of their wages and a further 33 weeks at a reduced amount. If you are self-employed, you may also be entitled to a maternity allowance from the government. Up-to-date guidance can be found at *gov.uk/employers-maternity-pay-leave*.

The UK government also now offers shared parental leave (SPL) which gives more choice in how two parents can care for their new baby. Parents can share up to 50 weeks of leave and up to 37 weeks of pay between them. This also applies to people who become parents through adoption.

When you notify your employee of your pregnancy, they must conduct a risk assessment, identifying any risks and adjustments that they may need to make to your working environment or hours. It could be that you usually work long days on your feet and these hours are reduced, or that you are given extra breaks throughout the day. If there are any hazards at work that may affect a pregnancy, this must be taken into consideration too. Employers are also legally obliged to allow you to have paid time off to attend antenatal appointments, including ultrasound scans.

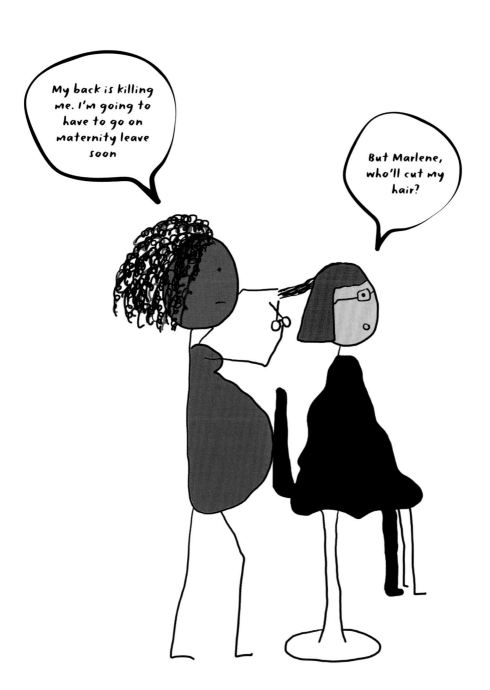

Group B Strep

Group B Streptococcus (GBS) is a bacterium which is carried by 20–40 per cent of adults, most commonly in the gut, and for up to 25 per cent of women who carry GBS, they have it in the vagina.

In most cases, there usually aren't any symptoms or side-effects, however GBS can occasionally cause infection, most commonly in newborn babies, sometimes in adults and, very rarely, during pregnancy and before labour. If it's not treated, GBS can increase the health risks to baby during birth and infancy.

In the UK, GBS is not routinely tested for on the NHS, but it can be picked up via a urine test or swab taken for other reasons. If the result is positive, antibiotics can be given in labour to prevent transmission to the baby.

There has been a lot of discussion regarding the reliability of GBS testing in pregnancy, as some people may test positive during pregnancy but negative in labour, and vice versa. This would mean some women receiving unnecessary antibiotics and some women missing out on them when they are needed. The best way to accurately test for GBS is during labour, but this hasn't been done historically due to the length of time it takes for results to come back.

A rapid test for use in childbirth has been manufactured but at the time of writing it is not readily available on the NHS or recommended for use by NICE (National Institute for Health and Care Excellence). In the UK you can pay for a private test during pregnancy but remember the result may not indicate your GBS status at birth as its presence in the vagina can come and go.

For more info on GBS and testing, visit *gbss.org.uk.*

Preparing The Mind And Body For Birth

No one can predict how your birth will go or what your experience will be like, but there are things you can do to prepare your mind and body for the big day.

Giving birth affects the body physically, so it's important to prepare so that you are in the best of physical health. Mental preparation is equally important, as the power of the mind will have a huge impact on your physiological responses. Have you ever considered that you can actually give yourself a birth mindset makeover during pregnancy?

I often tell people about my '70/30 birth rule'. I believe that 30 per cent of a birth experience is influenced by things you can't necessarily control, i.e. pre-existing medical factors, e.g. the position of the baby. The remaining 70 per cent of the birth experience is actually guided by things that can be controlled: environment and support, mindset, labour and birth positions, knowledge and confidence, physical preparation and wellness.

Let's begin by talking about physical preparation. If you actively prepare your body for labour and the birth of your baby, you have the potential to improve strength and stamina, increasing your overall likelihood of a better experience.

Overleaf are five ways you can help your body to prepare for the big day.

1. Keep mobile

Daily light exercise such as walking is a simple but effective way to keep fit, benefiting your body by improving your strength and endurance, particularly if you walk for at least twenty minutes per day. Walking in the fresh air is also a great way to clear your mind of stresses that may have built up throughout the day. Other forms of exercise you could try include yoga and swimming: yoga is great for improving core strength, and swimming can help with reducing swelling that may occur, particularly in your feet and ankles.

2. Use a birthing ball

Birthing balls can be used in pregnancy as well as in labour. When you're at home, rather than sitting on your sofa, try sitting on a birthing ball with your legs open slightly past your shoulders, rotating your hips in a figure of eight. This can prevent backache and also help open your pelvis, encouraging the optimal position for the baby to settle into.

3. Perineal massage

Regularly massaging the perineum (the skin between the vagina and anus) in the last 4–6 weeks of pregnancy is known to reduce the rates of perineal trauma and episiotomies. There is a lot of research and evidence to support this (you can start by looking on *evidence.nhs.uk*). It's really easy to do yourself, using a natural oil such as olive or coconut oil. If you find that your bump gets in the way, try asking your partner to help you.

Follow these steps to perform a perineal massage:

1. Ensure your hands are washed and you are in a comfortable position. This can be sitting, with one foot up on a stool or bath, or lying down if it's more comfortable.
2. Apply some natural oil suitable for the vagina, i.e. olive or coconut, to your thumb and perineal area.
3. Insert your thumb into your vagina approximately 3.8cm. Your thumb should be pressed downwards.
4. Using your thumb, apply pressure downwards, towards your rectum. Continue with this pressure, making a U-shape with your thumb from left to right. Imagine a clock pendulum swinging from 3 o'clock to 9 o'clock. As you do this, you may feel some stretching in the perineal area but it shouldn't hurt.
5. Continue massaging the area for three to five minutes.

Massaging your perineum at least three times a week can really make all the difference!

4. Eat dates

Eating healthily during pregnancy can help prevent complications further down the line, but did you know that there are specific foods that can increase your chances of having an easier and shorter labour?

There are tonnes of articles and information available on what snacks to eat during labour, but actually if you are looking to have the best birth you possibly can, then the dietary work needs to start around 8 weeks before your due date. This is when you are building up the nutritional stores that will fuel your body with what it needs to labour effectively. You may well have heard about the benefits of dates in pregnancy (the ones you eat, not go on!) – there have been several small studies which suggest that dates may indeed contribute to a more positive, smoother, easier birth.

One study showed that women who ate six dates a day for the 4 weeks prior to their due date had *significantly* easier labours compared to the group that did not eat dates! In the study, a number of positive effects were noted including:

- Went into labour spontaneously.
- Faster, easier dilation.
- Intact membranes on arrival to the hospital.
- Avoided the use of synthetic oxytocin drip to augment the birth.
- Had shorter first-stage labour.

Another study showed that women who consumed dates in late pregnancy experienced faster cervical ripening (softening) and dilating.

A date smoothie

If you fancy trying dates in your third trimester, I would recommend making a smoothie – blitz six large pitted dates with some of your favourite fresh fruits: strawberries and apples work well.

5. Mind preparation and releasing stress

Much of the fear and apprehension surrounding birth stems from what we have seen in the media, or been told by other people regarding their own worst experiences.

When you think back to a time when you have watched birth on TV, it probably starts with a smiling woman busily minding her own business before her waters dramatically break all over the floor. She then grips her abdomen as she doubles over in pain, and her partner begins panicking, running mindlessly around the house trying to find their car keys, before he bundles her puffing and panting into the car.

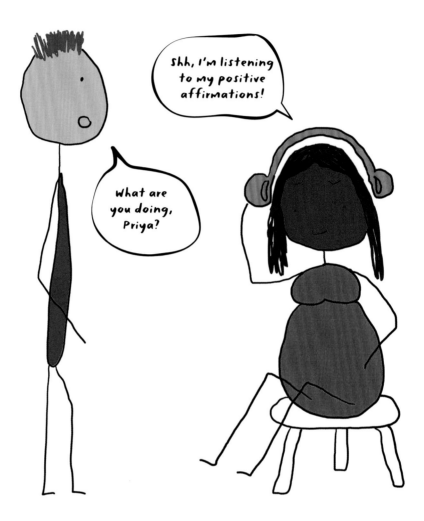

You may want to consider complementary therapies during pregnancy

These can be especially helpful if you are suffering from a lot of stress from work or family life. There is some evidence to support the use of aromatherapy, massage and acupressure during pregnancy. Always consult a qualified practitioner before undertaking any form of complementary therapy.

After speeding to the hospital and almost knocking over a few pedestrians along the way, the woman is quickly lifted into a labour room and has her legs put in stirrups before the doctor starts shouting at her to 'puuuush!' After screaming, sweating and cursing, the baby is finally born.

This is an unrealistic depiction of how birth is for most people.

When you are pregnant, some people feel compelled to tell you their traumatic birth stories. Now, while birth trauma is real, and should not be dismissed, the fact is that positive birth stories are shared less often. While someone telling you a negative birth story may feel like they are preparing you for all eventualities, what really ends up happening is that you begin to automatically associate birth with trauma, as there is no balance from the positive side. It's no wonder that so many people are fearful of giving birth.

You may have heard of the conscious and subconscious mind. The subconscious mind is like a filing cabinet full of every experience you have ever had. Your conscious mind is what you currently know and remember. If the majority of your experiences, thoughts and what you have learned about birth are negative, there's a stronger chance these will make it into your conscious mind when the time comes for you to have your baby.

So, what can you do to 'reprogramme' your mind? Avoid watching dramatic birth programmes that depict birth negatively. Watch positive births instead: you can find many on YouTube. When it comes to birth stories, if friends or acquaintances begin to tell you theirs, you can always interject and ask them to only continue if it's a positive one, or say you'd love to hear their story once you've had your baby.

Consider a hypnobirthing course to help you develop confidence and calmness, ready for the big day. Hypnobirthing encompasses a variety of tools and techniques such as visualisations, affirmations, breathing and scripts, to assist you in overcoming any fears you may have, while keeping you feeling focused and ready. Hypnobirthing can be useful in all birthing scenarios, including if your birth ends up requiring assistance.

Colostrum Harvesting

During pregnancy, your body starts to produce colostrum, the baby's first milk. This colostrum is full of goodness and is produced in very small amounts for the first few days after birth and may appear yellow, white or even clear.

Colostrum harvesting is a way in which to collect and store this first milk during late pregnancy, so that you have an additional supply in the event that baby needs it. Some people find it useful if baby initially has difficulty breastfeeding, or if the baby has low blood sugars and needs extra milk (this can sometimes happen with people who suffer with diabetes in pregnancy). There are many other scenarios where colostrum harvesting may be beneficial:

- Babies diagnosed with a cleft lip and/or palate, and other congenital conditions.
- Women with high blood pressure.
- Women who have had breast surgery in the past.
- Babies diagnosed with IUGR.
- Women having a planned caesarean.

Colostrum harvesting involves hand-expressing the milk and storing it in tiny syringes – these can be purchased online or may be available from your hospital (ask your care provider). For details on hand expressing, see page 190.

Once the colostrum is expressed, the syringes can be kept in the freezer and taken out to be given to the baby at a later stage. Colostrum harvesting is recommended only once you hit around 37 weeks' pregnancy, as nipple stimulation can cause contractions and there is a small risk of it initiating premature labour. It's highly unlikely (many people continue to breastfeed their toddlers while pregnant with no problems) but because it's a possibility, the following are advised not to express colostrum prior to 37 weeks' pregnancy:

- Those who have been told they are at risk of preterm labour.
- Those with a weak cervix or who have a cerclage (stitch) in place.
- Those carrying twins and higher multiples.

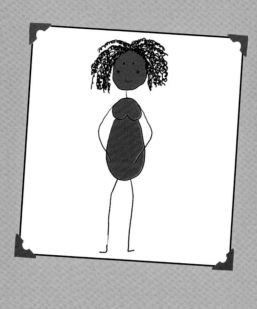

Your body carries extra blood when you're pregnant and this can cause your heart rate to increase so it beats about 25 per cent faster than usual.

When To Call Your Care Provider

Always trust your instinct if you feel something isn't quite right with your pregnancy, and get in touch with your midwife or GP.

The appropriate telephone numbers to call should be given to you at your first appointment with the midwife. If you are early in your pregnancy and have not seen anyone yet and have concerns, the hospital you're booked at should have an early pregnancy unit (EPU), which is there to provide support up to around 16 weeks' gestation.

Save all of the important contact numbers in your phone so that you are able to access them quickly and easily should you ever need to call.

Remember that there are some specific symptoms that should never be ignored, whatever stage you pregnancy is at. See opposite for a summary so you know what to look out for.

If you experience any of these symptoms, report them. Don't wait until the following day to get help and advice.

/ **REDUCED BABY MOVEMENTS**.
Call your maternity unit immediately if
your baby's movements have reduced,
slowed down or changed in any way. Don't
put it off until tomorrow.

/ **ITCHING**. Some itching over stretch
marks is expected as the skin stretches.
If the itching is persistent, however
– either mild or severe – particularly
on your hands and feet, it could be a
sign of the liver condition, intrahepatic
cholestasis of pregnancy (ICP). Other
signs include yellowing of the skin (not
always noticeable in darker complexions)
or yellowing of the eyes and mucous
membranes such as gums. Dark urine and
pale poo may also be noted. Your midwife
or doctor will be able to check for this by
performing a simple blood test.

/ **VISUAL DISTURBANCES AND/
OR SEVERE HEADACHES**. If you are
seeing 'floaters' or flashing lights, have
blurred vision and/or a severe headache,
these could be signs of pre-eclampsia.
Epigastric (chest) pain is also a symptom.

/ **SWELLING (OEDEMA)**. Sudden
swelling, particularly of the face, can be a
sign of pre-eclampsia. Swelling localised to
one area of the leg can be a sign of a blood
clot called deep vein thrombosis (DVT).

/ **ABDOMINAL PAIN**. At the end of
pregnancy, around your due date,
abdominal cramping is expected as a sign
of labour (see page 115). However, severe
abdominal pain that occurs suddenly, or
that is persistent, needs investigating so
call your care provider for advice.

/ **PRETERM LABOUR**. If you go into
labour prior to 37 weeks, it is classed
as 'preterm' or 'premature'. The main
sign of this happening is strong,
regular contractions which may feel
like menstrual cramps in the abdomen,
thighs or back to start with, and will get
stronger over time. Doctors may be able
to halt preterm labour in some instances,
depending on your gestation, labour stage
and other risk factors. Call the maternity
unit straight away if you think you may
be in preterm labour or if you think your
waters may have broken.

/ **PERSISTENT VOMITING**. If you are
vomiting so much that you are unable to
keep down fluids, you need to contact your
maternity unit so that they can assess
you in hospital. They may give you fluids
via an intravenous drip to prevent you
from becoming dehydrated. (Dehydration,
if untreated, can ultimately cause kidney
damage.)

/ **FEELING UNWELL**. Pregnancy
can often take it out of you and leave
you feeling drained of energy at times.
If you begin to feel really unwell, have any
dizziness, raised temperature or confusion,
seek advice from your care provider straight
away.

/ **VAGINAL BLEEDING**. While a bit
of brown/pink spotting is often normal
in early pregnancy, and may not be a
cause for alarm, seeing fresh, bright red
blood is not. If you experience vaginal
bleeding at any stage, whether or not
it's accompanied with abdominal pain,
contact your maternity unit for advice.

Practical Preparation For Welcoming Your Baby:
what will you need?

The list opposite covers everything you will want to consider buying for your baby, and for your recovery postnatally. If you want to know what to pack in your birth bag for the birth centre or hospital, or what to prepare for a homebirth, see pages 164–167.

Postnatal preparation tip

Spend the last couple of weeks before your due date cooking extra portions of meals and freezing them. That way, when you are home with baby, neither you nor your partner will have to worry about cooking for a while.

Things to have ready for baby's arrival	Optional
Clothing • Short-sleeved bodysuits x 15–20 • Long-sleeved onesies (babygro) x 15–20 • Hats x 5 • Scratch mittens x 4 • Cardigans x 5 • Outdoor/winter suit (*if applicable*) x 1	**Clothing** • Cute clothes (*dresses/trouser outfits etc.*) • Socks (*not needed if baby is wearing onesies with closed toes*)
Feeding • Burp/muslin cloths x 10 • Bibs x 20	**Feeding** • Breast pump • Breastmilk storage bags • Bottles and sterilising equipment • Formula (*if deciding to formula feed*) • Nursing pillow
Sleeping • Crib and bedding: mattress, waterproof cover and fitted sheet • Baby sleeping bag x 2 (*choose a temperature-appropriate tog*)	
Hygiene • Nappies • Cotton wool balls/water-based wipes • Soft cotton towels	**Hygiene** • Baby bath • Wedge-style bath support seat • Changing mat/station • Barrier/nappy-rash cream
Travel • Travel bag (*can be a simple rucksack*) • Pram • Car seat	
Accessories/Other • Blankets x 3 • Nail clippers	**Accessories/Other** • Swaddle wrap • Baby sling • Baby rocker
Postnatal recovery • Sanitary pads • Old/disposable knickers • Nursing bras • Breast pads • Nipple cream	**Postnatal recovery** • Perineal relief spray • Belly support belt • Paracetamol

Birth

In This Chapter

Labour and birth is not a one-size-fits-all!

We have explored what to expect during pregnancy, what's normal and what's not, along with tips on creating the best you, both physically and mentally, in preparation for the big day. This chapter will now fill you with knowledge about the birth process.

Share this information with your birth partner and use it to help you choose and write your birth preferences (see pages 102–103). Labour and birth are unique to everyone: although the information in this chapter will give you an overview of what birth looks and feels like in general, every labour and birth is an individual experience.

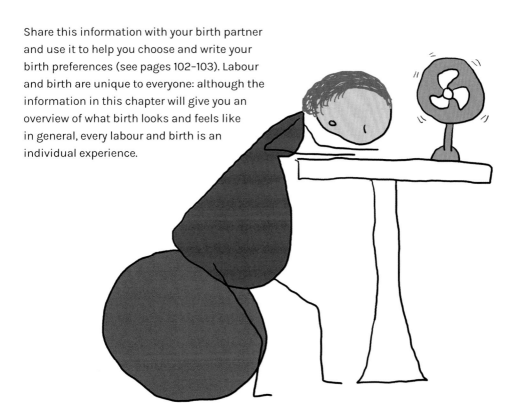

Factors That Can Affect The Birth Experience

We are mammals.

Yep, that's right – mammals, similar to the polar bears that live in the North Pole or the dingoes that roam the plains of Australia.

Mammals are designed to give birth with little to no assistance and to repeat the process several more times during the fertile life-span of the animal. Some mammals, however, need assistance, and this is where the vet steps in to assist or – for humans – the obstetrician.

Every woman and birthing person on Earth will have a unique childbirth experience. No two women will share a tale and no two pregnancies are the same. All four of my births have been totally different and, rather than compare them, I actually used my earlier experiences to shape my future ones into the births that I wanted.

There are five main factors which can have an impact on the ease and length of labour, and the overall birth experience:

1. Number of previous children.
2. Genetics.
3. Fitness and health.
4. Interventions.
5. Environment and mindset.

1. Number of previous children

It's no secret that if you have had a baby vaginally before (or at least laboured to some extent) then your next vaginal birth is more likely to be easier and shorter. The cervix seldom returns entirely to its pre-pregnancy state after giving birth, and the uterus has a great form of muscle memory. The shape of the uterus also changes after having a baby, going from pear-shaped to apple-shaped. All of this combined usually makes the cervix contract and dilate faster, requiring less effort.

Most second-time mothers I have cared for in labour have found the birth much more rapid and straightforward than their first.

2. Genetics

To an extent, genetics can play a role in your birth experience. The type of pelvis, for example, varies from woman to woman. There are four basic types of female pelvises and these are classified according to the shape of the pelvic brim or inlet. Did you know that pelvis is not a rigid structure? It is, in fact, an elastic system of bones that can stretch and widen as required. It is very flexible at the joints as it needs to open wide during labour. It is thought that the female population generally share mixed types of pelvises, but the four main types are:

- Gynaecoid.
- Android.
- Anthropoid.
- Platypelloid.

The gynaecoid is the most common pelvis, and platypelloid the least common. Some pregnant women become concerned that their babies won't be able to 'fit' through their pelvis. It is unlikely you will know what type of pelvis you have but be reassured that, regardless of its shape, most babies are able to fit through most pelvises. You cannot look at someone and determine that they will have trouble birthing based on their physical stature or abdominal size.

3. Fitness and health

Women who exercise and eat well during pregnancy are more likely to have a positive birth experience. In one Spanish study (source: see page 27), a cohort of around 500 women was divided into two groups. The first were led in sessions of moderate exercise by a professional three times per week. The remaining women had no intervention, just routine education about nutrition and physical activity during antenatal appointments. During the birth, there was quite a difference. The first stage of labour – the period where the cervix dilates to about 10cm – was an average of 53 minutes shorter for women in the exercise program. It wasn't just the first stage of labour that was affected: the women who exercised also had a slightly shorter second stage (pushing the baby out).

4. Interventions

Interventions during labour and birth can affect the outcome and experience a woman has. Interventions can include

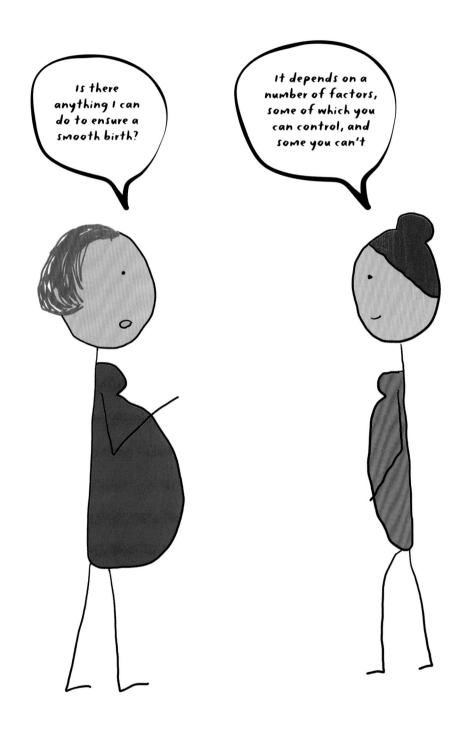

things like epidural anaesthesia, induction of labour, assisted births, caesareans, and amniotomy (artificially breaking the waters).

Some interventions are medically necessary to save the life of mother and/or baby, or to reduce the likelihood of long-term problems. An example would be someone who has developed severe pre-eclampsia during pregnancy; because the only cure known is for the baby to be born, an induction of labour may be recommended as the risks of remaining pregnant outweigh the risks of induction.

Some interventions can affect the physiological birth process, often leading to further interventions. The risks and benefits of any intervention should always be weighed up before making an informed decision.

5. Environment and mindset

Birth is more likely to go smoothly if you are in an environment that makes you feel safe and calm. Your birth setting can really impact how your uterus responds to labour and helps it progress.

The brain is an amazing thing; it produces the 'fight or flight' response, also known as the acute stress response, when it senses danger. This means the brain releases more of the stress hormones adrenalin and cortisol. These hormones slow down digestion, speed up the heart rate and move blood towards the major muscles in preparation for fighting or running. The essential muscle for childbirth, the uterus, gets left out and this can effectively stall labour.

Your mindset surrounding birth is very important, as fear of the unknown can hinder the birth in the same way. If the uterus is restricted of blood, delivering essential hormones, it can tense up, causing more pain. The increased pain causes more fear and distress, leaving a never-ending cycle of fear-tension-pain. The environment includes those that are supporting you during your birth; partners and healthcare professionals. If you feel supported and your wishes heard, you'll be more likely to release the positive labour-enhancing hormones. Having dim lighting, your own music and other comforts such as a blanket or pillow from home, may help you to feel more relaxed too.

What Is A Positive Birth Experience?

Contrary to popular belief, giving birth vaginally, at home, in water with no analgesia, and no perineal tears within four hours, is not the definition of a positive birth experience. Of course, for many that would be an ideal scenario, but a truly positive birth is actually subjective – one in which the mother is left feeling respected, heard, supported and happy about her experience.

Two reflections on the birth experience

Simone had an emergency caesarean, but was treated with utmost care during her experience, was able to make informed choices, had plenty of support postnatally, had her birth partner supporting her throughout, and felt she had prepared herself during her pregnancy for any eventuality. Simone reflects on her birth positively, even though it was not her plan to have an emergency caesarean.

Lucinda had a long labour. She gave birth vaginally eventually, but with the assistance of forceps. Lucinda has negative thoughts surrounding her birth as she didn't feel that she made any real informed decisions. She didn't feel particularly supported by her birth partner either, so the recovery afterwards was very hard. She doesn't have any positive memories about her birth.

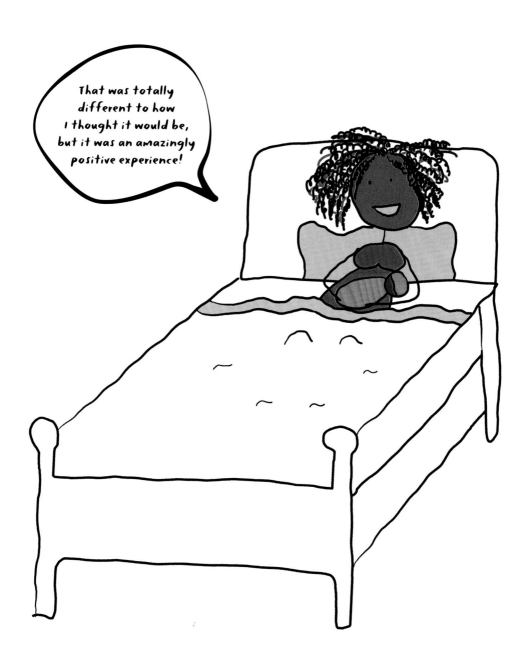

Birth Choices

Through every step of your pregnancy, birth and postnatal journey, you are in control of all aspects of your care. Any decisions on your plan of care, treatment or interventions are ultimately made by you.

Informed choice: understanding your options and making decisions

In the UK, women and birthing people have a right to safe and appropriate care that respects their choice, dignity, privacy and confidentiality, being free from discrimination or inequality.

You are well within your rights to question any care plan that a doctor (or any other health professional for that matter) has suggested for you. If an induction of labour has been suggested, for example, a doctor should always explain how it will benefit you and/or your baby.

If you are unsure, use the **BRAIN** acronym to help you evaluate your options and make an informed decision.

- *B* – What are the Benefits of such intervention?
- *R* – What are the Risks of the intervention?
- *A* – Are there any safe Alternatives?
- *I* – What does your Intuition tell you?
- *N* – What will happen if we do Nothing?

Your informed consent must be given before any treatment, examination or investigation can begin. That includes, but is not limited to: blood tests, vaginal examinations, medications and assisted births, the only exception to this would be in the case of someone who is unable to consent – either because they lack capacity or are in an absolute emergency situation where they are physically unable to (for example, they are unconscious).

Remember: this is your pregnancy, your body and your baby. The ball is always in your court!

Writing Your Birth Preferences

Writing your birth preferences is a good way of documenting everything that you are hoping for during and after the birth of your baby. Some people call this a 'birth plan' but I tend not to use thisterm as 'plans' are made to be stuck to and birth is never that rigid!

I strongly recommend writing birth preferences, as your birth partner and care giver will then have a record of your wants and wishes when you are in labour without having to repeatedly ask you questions. Before writing your birth preferences, do as much research as possible. By reading this book, taking a birth class and talking with your midwife, you will have a better understanding of the labour and birth process, what to expect, and what your options are.

Start thinking about your birth preferences by around week 34. Once you've jotted down some ideas, take it with you to your next midwife appointment, so you can discuss it, ask questions and clarify any policies that the hospital or birth centre have. If you are planning a homebirth, you will likely have a homebirth planning meeting with the midwife anyway. You can ask if they have time to go over your birth preferences then.

So, what should you include? Start with basic details such as your name, birth partner's name, due date and any medical or pregnancy concerns listed at the top, then use the guide opposite to help you think about what else you might want to add.

To write your birth preferences, simply create a document on your computer then print a couple of copies, keeping them in your birth bag. If that's not possible, a handwritten one is fine. When you greet your midwife in labour, ask them to read your birth preferences – don't assume they will automatically ask you for them.

Things you might want to include in your birth preferences document

/ FOR A PLANNED VAGINAL BIRTH

- Your thoughts on the environment, i.e. lighting, privacy, birthing balls etc.
- Your thoughts on pain management, e.g. have you been practising hypnobirthing, would you like to try Entonox (gas and air) or have an epidural, or are you open to seeing how you feel at the time?
- Your feelings surrounding episiotomy
- Would you like to have an active third stage? (See pages 108–110.)
- If you are unaware of the sex of the baby, who would you like to announce it? Do you want to see for yourself?
- Your thoughts on optimal cord clamping (see page 113) and who you would like to cut the cord.
- Your feelings around student midwives being present. They can be invaluable to help and support you, especially if your assigned midwife is called out of your room briefly. They are always working alongside midwives who mentor them. You may prefer fewer people in the room though, and that is totally your choice.
- Any other post-birth wishes you want to include, such as skin to skin, feeding choice and the 'golden hour', all of which are explained in the Fourth Trimester chapter of this book.

/ FOR A PLANNED CAESAREAN

- Your environment. Would you like any specific music played? The hospital may be able to accommodate this – just ask in advance. The lights will need to be on so that the surgeons can see what they are doing during surgery, but they may be able to dim the lights slightly at the moment of birth so that your baby has a gentler transition to meeting you.
- You may be able to see your baby being born by lowering the screen and even catch your baby yourself. Discuss this with your doctor to see if they are happy to facilitate this.
- Skin to skin. It is possible to have immediate skin to skin time with your baby after a caesarean if the baby is placed a little higher, with the support of your birth partner or midwife. As long as there are no concerns regarding you or the baby, this shouldn't be an issue.
- Whether you want photographs in the theatre room of you, baby being examined, or both.

Where To Give Birth:
hospital, birth centre or home

Generally, in the UK, there are three options available to people who are deciding on where to have their babies: at home, in a hospital or in a birth centre.

If you are considered to have a straightforward pregnancy, any of these birth locations may suit you. For those with some medical conditions or complications, it might be advisable to give birth in hospital, where help from the obstetric team is available if required. This is a conversation that you should have with your midwife or doctor, to help you make the best decision for you. In UK hospitals, midwives care for women throughout labour and birth, with obstetric doctors only stepping in to assist if an issue arises.

People who give birth at home or in a unit run by midwives (birth centre) are less likely to need assistance such as forceps or vacuum (sometimes called 'instrumental delivery'). As birth centres and homebirths are not attended by doctors, epidural anaesthesia is not possible. If you decide on a birth in one of these locations and then opt for an epidural, you will have to transfer into hospital. It's worth noting, though, that people who give birth at home or in birth centres are often more relaxed in these environments, making birth smoother and the need for an epidural less likely.

/ ARE HOMEBIRTHS SAFE?
For first-time mothers, homebirth slightly increases the risk of adverse outcomes for the baby – 5 in 1,000 for a hospital birth and 9 in 1,000 for a homebirth (according to figures from the NHS for 2020).

For women having their second or subsequent baby, a planned homebirth is just as safe as having your baby in hospital or a midwife-led unit. This is generally because having a straightforward birth first time around means that subsequent births are more likely to go the same, if not smoother.

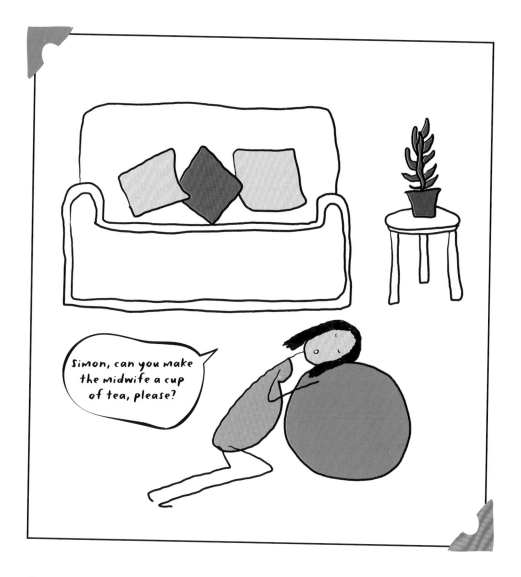

/ WHAT ABOUT BIRTH CENTRES?

These are facilities that are sometimes freestanding but are often attached to a hospital. This makes transferring into hospital easier if an issue arises. A birth centre is run by midwives and is usually a relaxed environment with minimal medical machinery, which helps with that 'home from home' feel. Birth centres will often have pools for water birth. Many units will offer virtual tours on their website so do ask if you would like to access one.

Wherever you choose, the place should feel right for you. You can change your mind at any point in your pregnancy.

Your Birth Environment

Environment is a key factor in the birth experience and outcomes. A woman needs to feel comfortable in the place that she is to birth her baby, be that at home, in a birth centre or in a hospital. Most low-risk women can be supported to give birth either at home or in a birth centre if they wish.

Being relaxed and comfortable during labour enables release of the feel-good hormones which aid the birth process. If you are in a constant state of fear and anxiety when you are in labour, the birth can be hindered due to the acceleration of adrenaline and suppression of endorphins and oxytocin. Choosing the best place for you to give birth is absolutely paramount in working towards having a positive experience, and choosing the best birth environment isn't limited to the place of birth. Considerations of the following can also be made:

- *Lighting* – Do you want the lights low to help create a relaxed mood?
- *Music* – Is there access to a music-playing device or can you bring your own in?
- *Birth partners* – Who will be supporting you? Your partner, mother, doula? Does the hospital or birth centre have a policy on birth partners?
- *Birth aids* – Will you have access to labour and birth aids such as the birthing ball?

Being able to remain as mobile as possible during labour will also help with the normal physiological birth process. If you are upright, the baby's head puts pressure on the cervix to help with dilatation. In addition, if you are moving around, the pelvis is able to flex and shift better so that the baby can negotiate it freely. If you are stuck lying flat on a bed the process can take more time. Most women find that during the active stage of labour lying still through contractions is uncomfortable. By simply standing or kneeling through contractions, you are able to rock your hips through each contraction and this freedom of movement can make you feel much more comfortable.

Stages Of Labour And Birth

Labour and birth is broken down into three stages:

STAGE 1 – Latent, Active and Transition

STAGE 2 – The Birth of Baby

STAGE 3 – Placental Delivery

What causes labour to start?

No one really knows what prompts labour to begin, but there are a few theories. Some suggest that when the baby's lungs are fully developed late in pregnancy, it triggers a response in the maternal system to begin labouring. Others hypothesise that the pituitary gland is responsible; it secretes higher levels of oxytocin when the baby is fully developed, which could be a trigger for labour.

The uterus and cervix are amazing organs that work together to ensure labour flows well. The uterus, which is made up of myriad muscle fibres, has to contract efficiently to shorten and dilate the cervix, allowing the baby to pass through. If contractions are not strong or frequent enough, the cervix will not dilate sufficiently, hindering the process. This can result in a very long early labour, or one that stops and starts over time, without any significant dilatation.

STAGE 1:
Latent and active

The first stage of labour and birth is broken
down into two stages – **latent** (often referred
to as 'early' or 'prodromal') and **active**
(sometimes called 'established'). Confusing,
right? Let me explain.

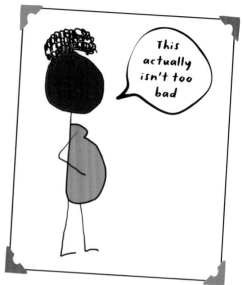

/ **LATENT PHASE**. The latent phase of
labour is when the cervix is in the process
of dilating up to roughly 4cm. Pre labour,
the cervix is a firm tube around 3cm long
and is closed at either end. The internal
opening is attached to the uterus. Initially
the cervix begins to soften in response to
prostaglandin hormone increase.
Contractions begin and continue to shorten
and dilate the cervix. This process can take hours or days for some women, depending
on many factors, including the ones I explained at the beginning of this chapter (see
pages 94–97). It often takes a long time as the uterus is busy trying to coordinate itself
to contract efficiently!

Some people, however, appear to completely miss the latent phase of labour and will
only notice they're in labour when the contractions are coming fast and the cervix is
already dilated to at least 4cm. In these situations, it's likely that the very early stage
wasn't recognised due to it happening quickly or the woman being so preoccupied with
her day that she didn't notice! This can happen with subsequent births, particularly if
the baby is well engaged into the pelvis and in an optimal position.

/ **ACTIVE PHASE**. The active labour begins when the cervix is around 4cm dilated
and the uterus is contracting at least every three to four minutes. This stage lasts
on average between eight to twelve hours for first-time mums and around five hours
for subsequent births.

The cervix needs to dilate to about 10cm to allow the baby's head to pass through.
Once active labour establishes, the body works hard to get to this stage.

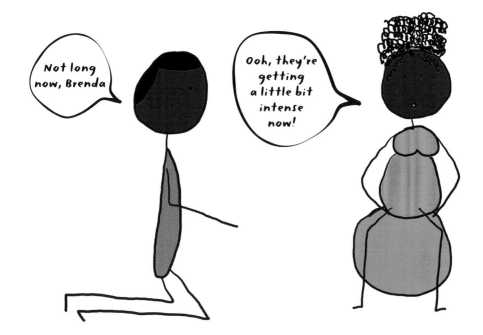

Transition

Transition is literally the final hurdle of labour. It is the period in which your cervix approaches full dilatation, and your baby starts to descend further down into the pelvis. This moment can feel quite scary and often women will later recall feeling slightly 'out of control'. It's not uncommon for women to vocalise their displeasure at this stage, saying they've had enough or want to go home; additionally, those who have previously coped well without an epidural may start asking for one now. This is often the most intense stage of labour and there is a lot of that stress hormone, adrenaline, surging around your body. Excessive adrenaline can hinder the early parts of the first stage, but when you are in transition, it gives you an extra boost of energy so that you can complete the last hurdle and birth your baby. The good thing, though, is that the transition phase is usually short-lived.

At some point through the transitional period, you should start to feel an urge to bear down (to 'push'). This is usually a sign that you are now fully dilated and baby is on the way. Sometimes, with a baby that is in a 'back to back' position, the urge may be felt earlier. If this is the case, your midwife may encourage you to try and resist pushing, as the pressure may make the cervix swollen if it's not dilated enough for the baby to pass through. Sometimes, adjusting your own position can help the baby to spin into a more optimal one – your midwife can assist you with this. The urge to bear down is stronger the lower the baby's head is in the birth canal, as it puts pressure on your rectum and

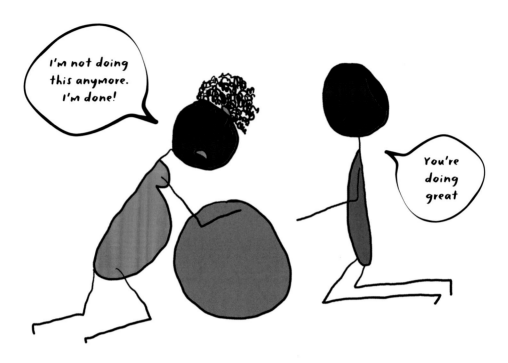

pelvic floor muscles, making you feel like you need to open your bowels. The transitional stage typically lasts five minutes to one hour but has been known to go on longer. Sometimes the urge to bear down is absent or not very strong: particularly with those who have opted for epidural anaesthesia, or with babies who aren't in optimal positions in the uterus.

When you hit the transition stage it's really important to stay focused. Maintain control and optimise oxygen intake by breathing slowly and deeply. Hold onto something that you can squeeze, such as the bed railing or door handle (without pulling it off), gas and air holder, or any other object that can't be broken! This will help you to focus and channel your energy.

I remember transition vividly with each of my births. I would know when it was happening as the contractions felt like they were non-stop, and I would start to feel like I couldn't go on anymore. What helped me, especially with my subsequent children, was focusing on controlling my breathing and knowing transition is the final leg of the race. It doesn't last long and it also helped to visualise my baby in my arms like the grand prize that babies are!

Your birth partner's support is crucial during this time, so here are some tips for them to read:

- Offer lots of encouragement, unless she prefers you to keep quiet. At this stage, eye contact and touch (if welcomed) may be a better form of communication.
- Breathe through the contractions with her to help her remain in control. Remind her to breathe slowly if she appears to start panicking.
- Be there, but give her space if she prefers. Not everyone likes being touched, especially in transition.
- Offer her ice chips/sips of water and a cold towel to mop her brow. If she feels cold, offer her a blanket.
- Transition isn't the best time for small-talk or jokes, so don't waste words. It will likely be more irritating than helpful.
- If her contractions seem to be very close together and she starts making grunting/pushing noises with no one in the room, it's best to call a midwife in at this stage. If in a hospital or birth centre, the call bell can be used.
- Remember that labour and birth is the most intense event someone can ever go through, so don't take it to heart if you're snapped at!

STAGE 2:
The birth of baby

The second stage of labour begins when you are fully dilated and ends when the baby is born. The process of actually birthing your baby, through the urges to bear down, can take anywhere from five minutes to a couple of hours. If it's your first baby, it's unlikely to be five minutes, as your pelvic muscles have never worked this way before.

The baby needs to rotate through the pelvis and work their way up and out by negotiating a curve in the birth canal. As your body pushes with each contraction, the baby makes more and more progress through this canal. Some people worry about opening their bowels as they are pushing. You may be glad to hear that pooing a little as you are pushing is extremely common – you wouldn't be alone if it happens to you. Chances are that if it does, no one would notice, apart from the midwife who would very quickly wipe it away.

Eventually, once the head is crowning, your midwife will support you to gently breathe the baby's head out. This approach helps to avoid significant vaginal and perineal trauma. Once the baby's head is born, usually the body is birthed with the next contraction. At this point, the second stage of labour is over. You will now be holding your precious baby while waiting for the next stage.

STAGE 3:
Placental delivery

The third stage now begins. After a while, the placenta, which has been nourishing your baby all this time, starts to detach from the lining of the uterus. This is managed in two ways: either active management – an injection of a synthetic oxytocic hormone is given into the thigh to speed up placental delivery, or physiological management – no injection is given and the placenta comes away when it's ready. With active management the placenta is usually expelled within a few minutes (but can take up to half an hour). With physiological management, this process can take longer (up to an hour). The choice as to how you would like to birth the placenta is totally yours.

Very occasionally, this stage doesn't happen as it should. If a placenta doesn't expel within an hour, it's referred to as 'retained' and may need to be manually removed by a surgeon in theatre under a spinal anaesthetic (if there isn't an epidural in already), as the risk of haemorrhage increases if a placenta is in the uterus for too long. Nothing can be felt as there will be a total block from the spinal anaesthetic/epidural. There are several reasons a placenta may not come away, including:

- The cervix closing before the placenta can come out – this can happen if the umbilical cord snaps after the birth.
- Placenta accreta – the placenta has embedded too deeply in the wall of the uterus.
- The uterus stops contracting so is unable to expel the placenta.

If the placenta is taking a little while to come out, your midwife may encourage you to change to an upright position and feed your baby if you're breastfeeding, as this can stimulate contractions. If a manual removal is recommended, this will be discussed with you fully first. Sometimes, a small amount of placenta remains in the uterus, which can also be a risk for haemorrhage and/or infection. This should pass naturally, but if not you may develop symptoms at home after the birth. These could include:

- Heavy bleeding, especially if it doesn't seem to be lessening.
- A sore and tender abdomen.
- Smelly vaginal discharge.
- Fever.

If you experience any of these, contact your maternity unit straight away for advice.

At some point between the birth of the baby and the delivery of the placenta, the umbilical cord is usually cut. If the placenta comes away quite quickly, the umbilical cord may not be cut until afterwards, especially if optimal cord clamping is being observed (see opposite).

Optimal Cord Clamping

Throughout pregnancy, your baby is connected to you via the umbilical cord, a narrow, gelatinous structure that passes blood and nutrients to the baby via the placenta. The cord has three vessels, one to carry blood to the baby and two to return blood and waste products from the baby back to the placenta.

Optimal cord clamping (OCC) is simply when the umbilical cord isn't cut immediately after the birth. It is also known as 'delayed' or 'deferred' cord clamping. Usually several minutes pass until the cord stops pulsating, at which point the cord is then cut. Delaying clamping the cord allows extra blood to be transferred from the placenta, increasing the amount of iron transferred to your baby. Iron is essential for brain development and infants with better iron levels seem to do better on tests of neurodevelopment later in childhood.

Babies who have had OCC are usually more stable at birth. When an umbilical cord is clamped straight away, there can be a sudden drop in blood pressure as blood is shifted towards the lungs as the baby takes their first breaths. OCC allows the extra blood that's in the placenta to travel into the baby, keeping the baby's circulatory system stable as it compensates for any drop in blood pressure.

There is a slightly increased risk of jaundice with OCC but it is usually mild and is usually resolved by plenty of feeding. If OCC is something you are interested in having after your birth, speak with your care provider or write it in your birth preferences.

Most care providers will delay clamping and cutting the cord now anyway, as it's recommended in the guidelines set out by the National Institute for Health and Care Excellence (NICE).

Tears And Episiotomy

Perineal tears are very common during childbirth, affecting around 85 per cent of birthing people.

The majority of perineal tears are small, requiring zero or minimal suturing and healing quickly after birth. First-degree tears affect only the skin and second-degree tears go deeper than the skin, affecting the muscle also. Third-degree tears affect the vaginal skin, tissues and muscles of the anal sphincter, while fourth-degree tears are the most serious, cutting through to the rectum. (Third-degree tears are not too common and fourth-degree tears are pretty rare.) Third- and fourth-degree tears can be problematic postnatally, as they take longer to heal and can cause postpartum incontinence, as well as causing other pelvic floor issues.

To reduce the risk of perineal tearing, you can try perineal massage in pregnancy (see page 80), and have a warm compress on the perineum during birth, as the head is crowning. Breathe your baby out gently and slowly, as if the baby comes out too quickly, you may be at risk of tearing more.

An episiotomy is a procedure where the perineum is cut with sterile scissors as the head is crowning during birth. Episiotomies should not be routine practice and should only be done with your consent if it is deemed necessary to expedite the birth, or if there is another medical reason to do so, for example in the case of a shoulder dystocia (the shoulder being stuck behind the pelvis), where a cut needs to be made so that the midwife or doctor can perform manoeuvres to free the baby.

Am I In Labour?
when to go to the hospital or birth centre

As you now know, labour tends to start gradually and lots of women won't even notice when it's in its early stages.

Contractions may not be obvious at first, but you might notice that you begin to feel a regular tightening/cramping of the lower abdomen or back that steadily gets stronger and more frequent. The contractions may start off feeling like a period-type pain and may also be felt in the groin and thighs. These are some signs that can indicate labour is imminent:

- *Having a 'show'* – A plug of mucus that has formed in the cervix to keep it sealed during pregnancy starts to break down and away through the vagina as the cervix softens and starts to dilate. This can happen several days before labour begins. You may notice some of this mucus as it is released from the vagina – it can appear as a large gelatinous lump that is yellow or brownish in colour.
- *Waters breaking* – This can occur before contractions but usually happens when contractions are already established. The membrane sac around the baby develops a hole and leaks amniotic fluid from the vagina. This may present as a trickle or a gush!
- *A feeling of 'knowing'* – Some women claim they knew that they were about to go into labour and started making preparations by 'nesting'. This involves suddenly getting ready for the baby to arrive, perhaps by an intense washing or sorting of baby clothes or even giving the house a spring clean out of nowhere!

The signs that a woman will feel will depend on several factors, including the position of the baby, whether or not you've had a baby before and your general wellbeing. If the baby is in a back to back position, you may feel most of the contractions in your back. If you have laboured before with a previous birth, you may find that the contractions intensify more quickly. Some women will lose their mucus plug well before labour starts and some won't. It varies from person to person. If you are experiencing regular contractions that are slowly intensifying and getting closer together this is a good sign, as it means that you are stepping closer to meeting your baby! However, if you find yourself in any of the following situations, you should inform your care provider immediately:

- If you are less than 37 weeks' pregnant and experiencing signs of labour.
- If your baby's movements are reduced – your baby should still be moving, even during labour.
- If you notice any vaginal bleeding – slight pink mucus/discharge (bloody show) is common in labour, especially if the cervix is dilating rapidly, but you should still mention it to your care provider.
- If you are feeling unwell, have a temperature and/or a rapid pulse.
- Your waters break and the colour is green or brown – this could be a sign that the baby has passed meconium (first poo) in the uterus and is occasionally a sign of foetal distress.

When should you get going?

You should call the birth centre/hospital/homebirth team if:

- You have been having strong contractions every four minutes (start of one contraction to the start of the next) for about two hours and each contraction is lasting one minute – think **4-2-1**.
- You think you are in labour and have a personal history of a precipitous (super-rapid) birth, even if you are not contracting as above.
- You are experiencing any of the causes for concern mentioned above.

If you are worried about anything at all, or feel you need support or advice, call your midwife. If you are less than 37 weeks' pregnant, call your care provider at the earliest opportunity.

Advice for keeping calm

- Practise relaxation techniques that are used in programmes such as hypnobirthing.
- Keep mobile. Moving around will help you to cope with the contractions, as well as assist in your progress.
- Practise slow, deep breathing.
- Try not to panic! If you are asked to go into the hospital or birth centre to be assessed, remember to collect your bag, notes, birth preferences and anything else you need. This could be a job for your birth partner.

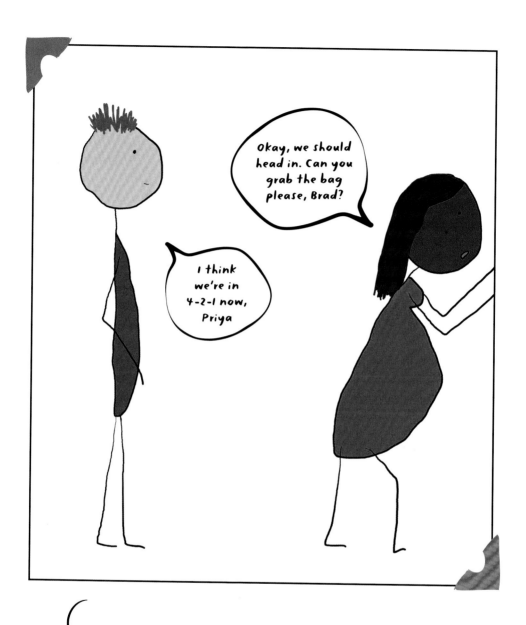

Remember, each contraction will bring you closer to meeting your baby!

Coping With Pre-labour

Prior to going into established or active labour, there is often a period of pre-labour. This is sometimes referred to as the 'latent phase', 'prodromal' or 'early labour'.

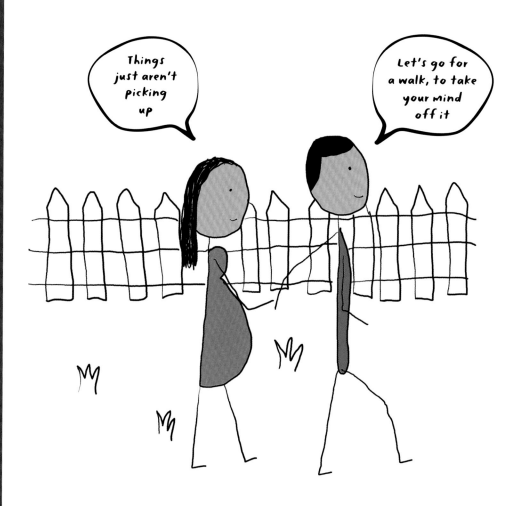

Some sources call early labour 'false labour', but this is not an accurate term: although this phase can be exhausting – lasting anywhere from several hours to several days – the contractions you may experience, even if they have a stop-start pattern, are likely to be making small but crucial changes to your cervix in preparation for established labour.

For some people, pre-labour can be an extremely frustrating time. You may experience contractions that are mild and irregular, and that drag on for what seems like forever. They may just stop for hours before re-starting, and they can have you wondering if you are ever going to meet your baby.

Annoyingly for many women in this position, they head to the hospital or birth centre too soon, only to be disappointed to find out that the cervix has not dilated, or is not as dilated as they had hoped. In most cases changes have been occurring, which is a step in the right direction, but the body is going at its own pace, which is totally okay. Even if it's not as quick as the birthing person had hoped!

A long pre-labour is more likely to occur in someone who has a baby that is in an OP position (back to back), other malpresentation, or who is tense and anxious. The best thing to do if you are experiencing a long, drawn-out pre-labour is to keep as busy and distracted as you possibly can. You can try the following:

- **Go for a walk with your birth partner.** The fresh air will do you good, and walking will help the pelvis to open for the baby's head.
- **Try a warm bath.** The warm water can be relaxing, helping you to feel calm.
- **Watch a comedy.** Nothing is better at generating those feel-good hormones than laughter!
- **Listen to music.** They say music is medicine. Listening and even dancing to music can help pick you up a little during the early stages.

- **Use a birthing ball.** Sitting on a birthing ball while rocking your hips side to side, or bouncing, can help.
- **Urinate frequently.** A full bladder may affect the uterus' ability to contract effectively, and may hinder the baby's head going down into the pelvis.
- **Rest.** Sometimes having a good sleep, if you can, can relax you enough to get things going. Having a lower back and shoulder massage prior to resting will give you that additional 'feel-good factor'.

Not everyone experiences a long pre-labour. The uterus has two segments, the upper and lower. Both segments have muscle fibres that must act together to create effective contractions which will dilate the cervix. Effective contractions coupled with an optimal foetal position (with the baby well-engaged into the pelvis) may make pre-labour shorter or non-existent. This is also true for women who have birthed before, due to muscle memory.

When And If Your Waters Break:
what to do and what to look out for

Your baby is suspended in a sac of amniotic fluid throughout pregnancy. This fluid is made up mostly of your baby's urine, but also includes antibodies, hormones and nutrients to support your baby's wellbeing. An unborn baby will regularly swallow this fluid and pee it out again.

For the baby to enter the world, the membrane sac that contains them needs to rupture. In most cases, this happens at some point during labour, with some of the amniotic fluid leaking out of the vagina, an event known as 'waters breaking'. Some waters don't break at all and the baby is born in the sac. This is also known as being born 'en caul'.

For around 10 per cent of pregnant women, waters break before labour starts (i.e. before the onset of any contractions). The good thing is that, in most cases, labour begins within a few hours of this happening. If you suspect your waters have broken, pop on a sanitary pad and check the colour of the fluid. Amniotic fluid should drain clear or slightly straw-coloured. If it appears brown, green, pink or red, you will need to let your care provider know straight away. Brown/green fluid can be a sign of the baby passing meconium (first poo) in the womb. Much of the time this doesn't affect the baby at all, but it can cause problems in some cases if the baby inhales it during the birth. If the fluid is pink or red, that can signify a bleed coming from somewhere (potentially the placenta) that will need to be looked at.

If a lot of time passes after the waters break, without any sign of labour, there is an increased risk of developing a serious infection as the protective bag around the baby has now been broken. The overall risk of developing an infection is around 1 in 100 (1 per cent) for those whose waters have been broken for over twenty-four hours prior to labour, as opposed to 1 in 200 (0.5 per cent) for those who go into labour with their membranes intact. This still means that 99 per cent of women whose waters have been broken for over twenty-four hours won't develop an infection. Nonetheless, because of

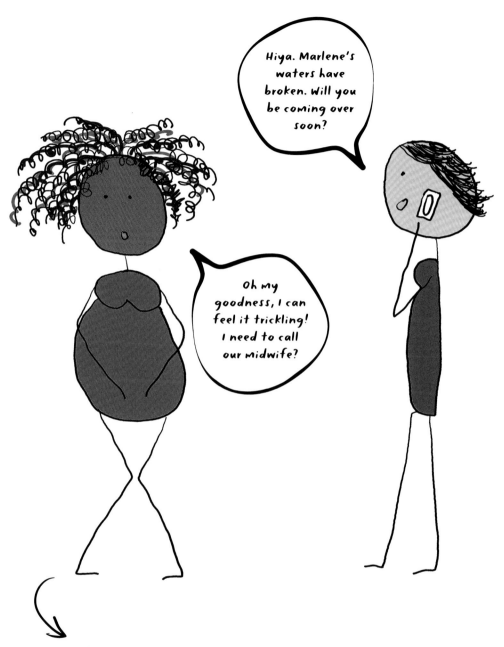

If you suspect your waters have broken, pop on a sanitary pad and check the colour of the fluid.

this increase in risk, care providers will offer an induction to kick-start your body into labour if there are no contractions. When they do this varies, but most hospital guidelines suggest around twenty-four hours after your waters have broken. If you decide you do not want an induction and would rather wait for labour to begin naturally, your care provider will advise you on keeping an eye out for signs of infection by checking your temperature regularly and monitoring your vaginal discharge/colour of amniotic fluid.

You will also be advised to avoid sexual intercourse, use sanitary pads only, not tampons, avoid public swimming baths and avoid the use of any cosmetics around your genital area, including perfumed soap or deodorising sprays. You can continue to shower and bathe normally. Keeping an eye on your baby's movements is also important. If infection is suspected, antibiotics may be given during labour.

Read on to the 'If labour slows down or stalls' section (pages 129–131), for things that you can do if your waters break but you are not experiencing contractions, to encourage labour naturally.

If you are under 37 weeks' pregnant and you think your waters have broken, call your care provider without delay. They will most likely advise you to go to hospital for further care as your baby is premature.

What are hindwaters and forewaters?

There is a lot of confusion surrounding hindwaters and forewaters. The forewaters are simply the collection of fluid in the sac in front of the baby's head, with the hindwaters being the part of the water-filled sac that sits behind the baby's body. Some people mention their hindwaters breaking but not their forewaters. Sometimes, your waters break, you feel a leak and are adamant it's not urine, only to be told at the hospital after being examined that the part of the bag of water in front of the baby's head is still intact. In these situations, the person has felt a hindwater trickle.

With hindwater leaks, these too can happen before or during labour. Often they may appear to be more of a trickle as the baby's head is plugging the cervix. You may even think you've peed yourself!

The pelvis is not a rigid structure. It is an elastic system of bones that can stretch and widen as required.

Vaginal Examinations In Labour

Vaginal examinations, also called cervical or internal exams, are commonly offered both prior to labour being induced, and to assess the progress of labour.

Vaginal examinations are conducted by feeling the position, length, consistency and dilatation of the cervix. The position of the baby's head in the pelvis can usually be felt, which helps give insight into the progression of labour.

The procedure is done by the care provider, who inserts two fingers into the vagina until the cervix is felt. It can be quite a daunting experience for some people, especially if you have never had a vaginal examination before, and what it feels like will depend on the individual. The position of the cervix needs to be taken into consideration, as a cervix that is very posterior will be more difficult to reach, potentially causing more discomfort.

If you think you are in labour as you have been having regular minute-long contractions for two hours – remember **4-2-1** (page 116) – a vaginal examination will be offered to check on the dilatation. An examination to confirm established labour is not always necessary and your informed consent must be gained first. Often, those who turn up to be assessed are clearly in established labour, and many midwives are able to recognise signs of this by seeing how the pregnant person is behaving, without needing to perform a vaginal examination.

Appearances can be deceptive, however. If you have practised hypnobirthing techniques, you may appear to be much calmer and focused than is typical. This can mislead some midwives into thinking perhaps you're not in established labour! For this reason, if you use hypnobirthing techniques in labour, always let the midwife know.

Another way a midwife may be able to tell how close you are to giving birth, is by assessing the appearance of a 'labour line'. This is a line of pigment that creeps up the back from the top of the buttocks. When it reaches a certain height, it usually means

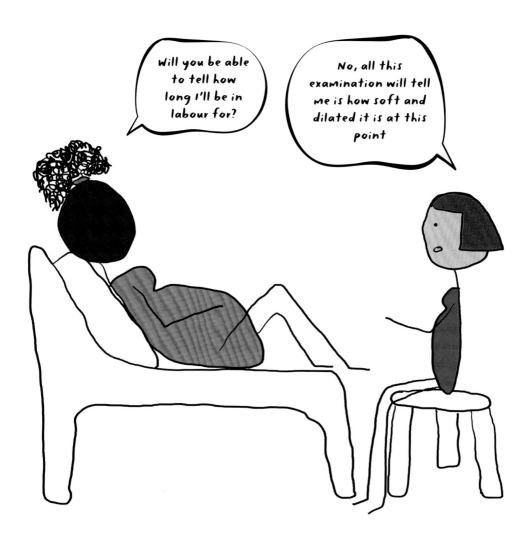

there is full dilatation. This line isn't visible in everyone. It can appear purple, red, brown/ black, grey or pink, depending on your normal complexion. Whether you have a vaginal examination or not is totally your call. You have a right to decline if you wish.

The rate at which a cervix will dilate once in established labour varies from person to person. Some people will go from 3cm to 8cm in one hour, others will steadily dilate 1cm every two hours. When looking at progress, the whole picture needs to be considered, including your and your baby's wellbeing, the baby's position, and how you are coping.

Positions For Labour And Birth

During labour, many women will adopt different positions to help them get through. This often comes naturally, depending on the stage of labour and how much energy she has at the time.

It is best to remain mobile and as upright as possible during the early stages of labour – it is often assumed that sitting down on the bed is ideal, but this can potentially slow down labour and make you feel more uncomfortable. Adopting a balance between being mobile and resting is vital for progressing labour and maintaining sufficient energy for the birth.

Positions for labour

When you are mainly upright during labour, gravity helps provide pressure from the baby's head onto the cervix, encouraging strong contractions to push the baby down towards the birth canal. Upright positions include:

- Standing, legs hip-width apart, hands on a table, wall or birthing partner, and gently rocking hips from side to side.
- Sitting/bouncing on a birthing ball.
- Kneeling over a bed or sofa.
- Standing, leaning on a birthing partner.
- Being in water which allows for upright labour and birth positions.

Some women complain of backache during labour, which is often due to the baby lying with their spine against their mother's spine in the womb (known as posterior position). If you struggle with this, your partner could perform a 'hip squeeze' through each contraction, to help provide some relief: this involves them placing a hand on either side of your hips from behind and squeezing as if they are trying to make their hands touch. If the baby is lying in a sub-optimal position, or their head is out of alignment with the pelvis, this can cause labour to be slow as well as uncomfortable. Lying in an exaggerated lateral or open-knee chest position for around half an hour is renowned for encouraging babies to rotate, expediting the birth.

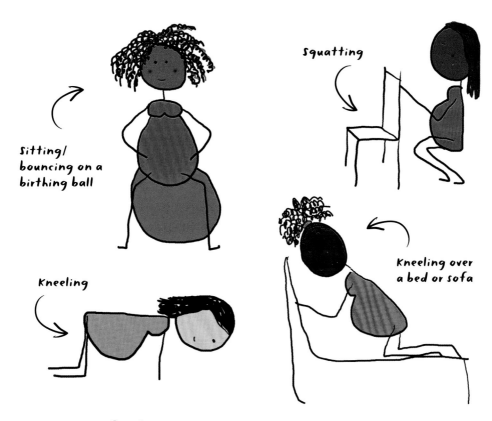

Sitting/bouncing on a birthing ball

Squatting

Kneeling

Kneeling over a bed or sofa

Positions for birth

During the birth, a variety of positions can be adopted. Being more upright tends to reduce the chance of needing an assisted birth via either forceps or suction: the pelvic outlet is wider, the uterine muscles can contract effectively, and pushing efforts are easier. Kneeling, squatting and being on all-fours are fantastic birthing positions, and as well as experiencing the benefits listed above, you are able to see and pick up your baby immediately after the birth.

If you have an epidural, lying flat on your back should ideally be avoided as it can slow down labour and make your blood pressure drop. Some epidurals enable you to mobilise into different positions, aiding the birth process. A study carried out in 2017 by the Royal College of Midwives concluded that side-lying when pushing in women who had 'low dose' epidurals (lower-strength ones in which there was not total leg numbness) reduces the risk of the birth needing to be assisted with instruments or surgery. If lying on one side affects the distribution of the epidural, try to remain sitting as upright as possible. Better still, when the anaesthetist arrives, ask them if they can administer a 'mobile' epidural that doesn't affect the use of your legs. This will allow you to adopt a range of positions while still benefitting from the anaesthetic.

Breathing Techniques

Deep, controlled breathing throughout labour and birth will help you to remain in control, as well as allow your uterus to work most effectively. In an approach called hypnobirthing, 'up breathing' is used during the first stage of labour and 'down breathing' is used during the birth (for more on hypnobirthing, see page 139). You can practise these breathing techniques at home during your pregnancy in preparation for the big day.

Up breathing

Relax your shoulders and arms. Blow out, then gently breathe in through your nose to the count of five, filling your lungs with air. Count slowly 1...2...3...4...5. Pause for a split second then exhale through the mouth to the count of six. Release the breath naturally. 1...2...3...4...5...6. Everyone has different lung capacity, so if you find it tricky, just breathe as slowly and deeply as you can, ensuring that the exhale is longer than the inhale. Controlling your breathing encourages oxygen to flow around your body which helps the uterus work effectively, promotes relaxation and distracts you during your contractions in the first stage of labour. Between contractions, allow your breathing pattern to return to normal. If you like, use visualisations along with the breathing technique, such as imagining a dial on the wall with a large hand set at 10. Visualise the hand counting down slowly until it gets to 1. At this stage, the contractions should start wearing off. Practise up breathing for a few minutes each day. Encourage your birth partner to help by counting with you.

Down breathing

Once you have gone through the transitional phase and start getting an urge to bear down, down breathing can help guide your baby through the birth canal gently. You can practise this too – ideally when you are on the toilet, then the practice is productive! Relax your shoulders and arms. Take a short breath in through your nose and focus for a second. Exhale through the mouth to the count of eight, channelling your breath down through your body to your pelvic floor: this helps bring baby further down the birth canal with each contraction and breath. In the second stage of labour, you should feel your body starting to bear down involuntarily – the down breathing simply aids the process. You will probably notice that the contractions are more spaced out now: this is so that you conserve energy and catch your breath between each one.

If Labour Slows Down Or Stalls

So, you have found yourself in established labour. Your contractions have been coming regularly and your cervix has been dilating effectively. Suddenly things appear to slow down, contractions may appear to ease off and/or your cervix has decided to stop opening.

If labour slows down or stalls, it can be an extremely difficult and frustrating time, often causing further anxiety and the possibility of slipping into the fear-tension-pain cycle that I mentioned previously (on page 97). You'll be glad to know, though, that for the majority of people who experience a slowed or stalled labour, it's only a temporary glitch.

There can be a variety of reasons why things may slow down; perhaps the position of the baby is preventing them going down deeper into the pelvis, maybe oxytocin is being inhibited, which is having an effect on the strength of contractions, or there could even be an emotional stress causing labour to slow down or stall.

It's common for care providers to suggest giving you the synthetic form of oxytocin in a drip, to get the contractions going again, but this isn't always necessary, or helpful. The synthetic hormone used can cause quite strong contractions that are more intense than natural ones, often making it difficult to cope with. If this is offered, it's always worthwhile asking the question 'is there anything else we can try first?'. On the next page are a few things you could try, to hopefully avoid being in that scenario!

Think about changing your position

It's good to mobilise in labour and to remain as upright as possible, so if you have been lying down or have been in one position for a long time, try changing position. This can adjust your pelvis, and that adjustment may support your baby better, helping the cervix to dilate more. Doing lunges or squats may give baby the extra little nudge they need. If you are exhausted from walking around, lie down on your side with one knee raised. There are other positions you could try, too:

- Exaggerated lateral side-lying.
- Forward-leaning inversion (only do this under the watchful eye of your care provider. Avoid if you have high blood pressure, glaucoma or polyhydramnios).
- Kneeling, with bottom in the air (gently wiggling your hips from side to side in this position may help, too!)

Refer to *milescircuit.com* for a visual guide to these positions.

> Sometimes a little recovery and energy conservation is all that's needed to get things going again. Resting with your knees up, in foetal position, can help with the rotation and descent of the baby.

Try nipple stimulation

Nipple stimulation is known to produce uterine contractions, as it causes the release of oxytocin. If the contractions have slowed down, you can do this by rolling your nipples between your thumb and forefinger, or by using a breast pump if you have one to hand.

Change your environment

If the room is noisy, ask for things to be kept quiet. Dim the lights, check the temperature of the room if you can, request privacy if you need it, and even grab hold of your pillow from home. Environmental stimuli really can make all the difference.

By trying all of these things, the idea is that you will hopefully give your body and mind a helping hand to continue labour on the right path, without the need for intervention.

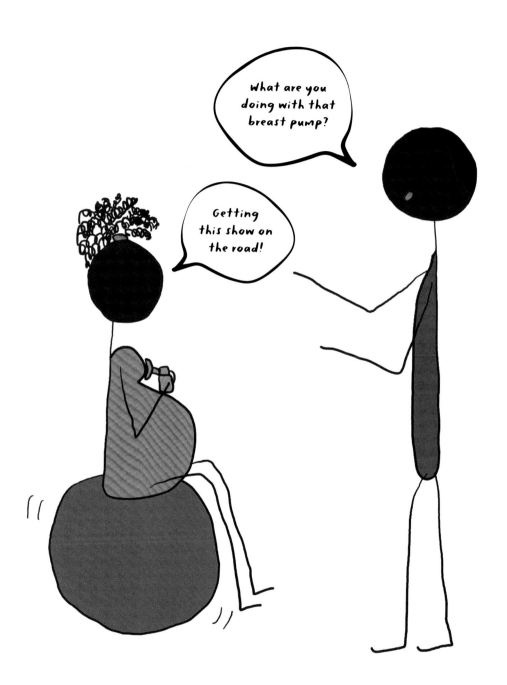

Membrane Sweeps

A membrane sweep, or stripping the membrane, is a drug-free way of encouraging labour when you are overdue, to avoid a medical induction. You do not have to have a membrane sweep if you don't want to.

So, how is a membrane sweep performed? The midwife or obstetrician puts a finger into the cervix and makes a circular or sweeping movement around the baby's head if it's low enough (or simply around the neck of the cervix). The point of it is to separate the sac surrounding your baby from the cervix. This can stir up some hormones to start softening and dilating the cervix and subsequently put you into labour. A membrane sweep can be uncomfortable, especially if the cervix is very posterior, and can also cause some light bleeding.

If the cervix is closed, a membrane sweep would not be possible and therefore ineffective. It is more likely to have an effect if you are past your due date as often cervical changes have already begun to occur and your body is more likely to be ready for labour anyway. A literature review published in 2020 suggested that going into spontaneous labour may be more likely with a membrane sweep but more evidence of certainty is needed.

Membrane sweeps aren't just offered as a way of avoiding a medical induction when you are past your due date. They are sometimes considered prior to an earlier induction for medical reasons, such as the case of someone who has agreed to an induction at 38 weeks due to pre-eclampsia.

The midwife has offered me a sweep

You can request more than one membrane sweep if the first doesn't work, or you don't have to have one at all! It's totally your call.

Induction Of Labour

An 'induction of labour' is when labour is brought on with the help of medical interventions.

There are a number of reasons why an induction might be offered, the most common one being that you're a week or so past your due date. There have been several studies and reviews into the outcomes of pregnancies that go beyond 41 weeks. Some of these studies have concluded that the stillbirth rate increases slightly after 41 weeks and others have shown no difference. The differing results in these studies make it extremely confusing for those who are deciding on whether to go ahead with a medical induction for being 'overdue'.

An alternative way to determine the real risk is to look at the entire population, rather than groups reviewed for studies. The MBRRACE-UK report (Mothers and Babies: Reducing Risk through Audits and Confidential Enquiries across the UK) provides statistics on UK stillbirth rates. Interestingly, the data collected in 2018 showed that of babies that were born between 37–41 weeks, there were 1.2 stillbirths per thousand.

The Office for National Statistics (ONS) also provides data on births throughout the UK, and in 2017 they published the stillbirth rates. The findings were similar to the MBRRACE report:

Gestation	Stillbirth rate per thousand births
40	1.03
41	1.03
42	0.96

Many factors determine when you'll go into labour, including genetics, ethnicity, height and overall health. While most babies are born spontaneously before 42 weeks, some are not.

Sometimes induction of labour is offered because of a medical need, meaning it would be riskier for you or your baby if you remained pregnant. Some of these reasons include:

- Pre-eclampsia.
- Uncontrolled gestational diabetes.
- ICP (intrahepatic cholestasis of pregnancy).
- IUGR (intrauterine growth restriction).
- Other maternal illness which puts you at more risk than the baby if you were to remain pregnant rather than give birth.
- Persistent reduced foetal movements.

Induction can be offered but you always have a choice. Get information from your care provider so you can make an informed decision. If you do not want an induction, discuss it with your care provider and review close monitoring in the final days of your pregnancy. Many uncomplicated spontaneous births have occurred at over 42 weeks' gestation.

What an induction involves

When considering what method to use, your care provider will perform a vaginal examination to assess the cervix and see how 'favourable' it is. If your cervix is closed, with no signs of any changes, the first step would be to insert a prostaglandin hormone in the form of a pessary (a tablet that goes into the vagina), or a gel behind the cervix. This is often enough to soften the cervix and kickstart labour, but it doesn't work for everyone and may require further doses. Usually, no more than three doses are given in a twenty-four-hour period. If the cervix starts to soften and dilate but there are no strong contractions, the next step would be for a doctor or midwife to break your waters vaginally with an amnihook. This can be enough to get labour going, but if not, a third step is introduced – the synthetic oxytocin drip. This drug brings on powerful contractions to help dilate your cervix. As this intervention makes the uterus contract in an unnatural manner, there is a small risk of baby not tolerating it well, so continuous foetal heart-rate monitoring is required. It can also sometimes cause the uterus to contract too much which can cause complications, so you will be monitored carefully.

Occasionally, a non-pharmacological method such as the foley balloon is used to dilate the cervix (for example, if you have previously had a caesarean and prostaglandins can't be used, due to a risk of your uterus rupturing). A doctor will place a catheter through your cervix with a balloon and the balloon is then filled with a saline solution which helps the cervix dilate. Induction of labour is an intervention known to increase the necessity of having a caesarean, but plenty of women have also had successful vaginal births via this practice. It's important to know that for many people, induction of labour can take a long time, sometimes days. There is also a chance that it may not work at all.

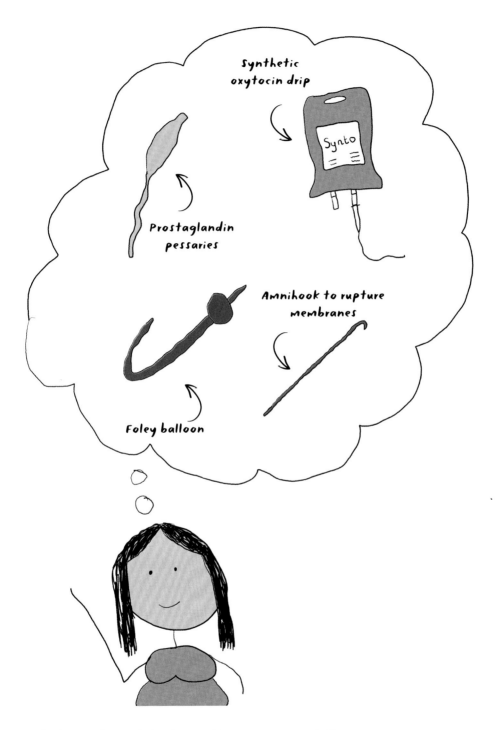

Synthetic oxytocin drip

Synto

Prostaglandin pessaries

Amnihook to rupture membranes

Foley balloon

For further reading on induction, see Resources on page 248.

Water Birth

If you are enjoying a straightforward pregnancy, a water birth might be an option to consider. Some women love it and others don't, but it's certainly a gentle way for baby to enter the world! If your pregnancy is complex, a water birth doesn't necessarily have to be ruled out. Discuss it with your midwife if it's something you would like to consider.

Many pregnant women find having a bath or shower comforting, and this feeling of relaxation in water can continue into labour. The buoyancy of water can feel really good and it's easier to move into any position that suits you. It is also thought that the water may set off an oxytocin surge, helping to increase the efficacy of contractions.

Some studies suggest that water birth can also shorten the second stage of labour. Most birth centres and some hospitals will have pools that you can use during labour and birth. You can also hire or buy a birthing pool to use at home if you wish. The midwife looking after you will be pretty hands off during a water birth, allowing you space to focus, relax and breathe!

You can usually get into the birthing pool at any point you like if you're having a homebirth, even during pre-labour if you feel it helps. In a hospital or birth-centre setting, it's more likely that you would be in established labour before you get into the pool. If at any stage you want to get out of the water, that's not a problem at all. Some women get in and then decide to get right back out again. (In fact, labouring in a standard bath but giving birth on dry land is another option to consider if a water birth is not available or possible.) When the baby is born in water, they are still receiving oxygen via the umbilical cord for a couple of minutes, so baby will be safe as they make their way up to the surface.

If your labour is induced, or if you have other complications with your pregnancy but still want a water birth, this is something you will have to discuss with your doctor or midwife. During a water birth, you should be able to use Entonox (gas and air), but will not be able to have an epidural. The use of opioid analgesia is also not recommended for use with a water birth, unless sufficient time has passed so that the effects have worn off.

During a water birth, the midwife will need to check the temperature of the water frequently and will offer intermittent heart-rate monitoring of the baby using a

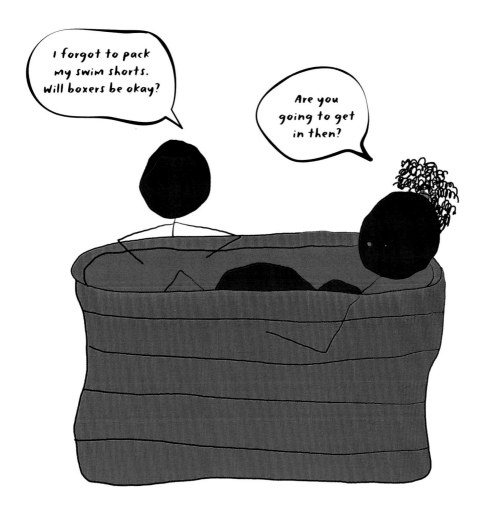

handheld Doppler (a small electronic device with a probe that detects the baby's heartbeat via your abdomen).

Some studies suggest that the likelihood of serious tears (i.e. third and fourth degree) may be significantly reduced by having a water birth but smaller, less significant tears (first or second degree) might be more common. The reduction in serious tears may be due to the fact that giving birth in the pool usually enables a better birthing position and also the warm water helps relax the perineum. The potential increase in minor tears may be due to the reduction in visibility for the midwife and being totally hands off, reducing her ability to provide perineal support if needed.

Some partners like to hop into the pool too, offering support as the baby is welcomed into the world. They just need to remember to pack swimming shorts or a swimsuit!

Pain Relief Options:
pharmacological and non-pharmacological

One of the biggest topics of discussion surrounding childbirth is pain and how to manage it. There is no denying that when a muscle cramps, it can hurt. The uterus is a muscular organ that behaves in the same way, but with more of a purpose than other muscles that cramp. You may find comfort in working with the pain, acknowledging its role in the progression of labour and considering it as positive affirmation that you are getting closer to meeting your baby.

The ways women remember labour pain differ vastly, with some giving it a 3 on a scale of 1–10 and others giving it a 10. How pain signals are processed varies from person to person, and will be affected by factors I have mentioned previously such as mindset, environment and physiological traits. It's good to know what options you have for managing the intensity of labour, whether it's pharmacological (medicines) or non-pharmacological (natural methods), so that you can choose what's best for you. You may not know what you want and that's okay: think of everything you are going to read here as a scale – you may want to consider natural, non-invasive forms of pain management first, and work your way up in labour if you feel you need to.

Non-pharmacological

/ **WATER**. Many women use warm water as a form of pain relief during labour. It acts in a similar way to using a hot water bottle on your abdomen if you suffer from menstrual cramps. Some women opt for a water birth, but many simply use water in a bath or birthing pool to ease contractions, then get out for the birth. If you can't access a bath or birthing pool, a warm shower can provide some relief. If you have back pain, aim the shower head on your lower back: this acts as a massage and staying upright may help with the natural transition of labour. You can also combine water with other forms of pain management such as Entonox and hypnobirthing. Water won't completely remove the discomfort of contractions but it can take the edge off.

/ **HYPNOBIRTHING**. As I mentioned on page 128, hypnobirthing is a form of managing pain through techniques designed to 'reprogramme' the way you view birth, by teaching you methods to remain calm, release fear, build confidence and 'hypnotise' yourself during labour so that you are less aware of any discomfort. This is done through a number of methods such as visualisations, scripted meditations, breathing, light-touch massage and developing 'triggers' with your birth partner. Hypnobirthing requires time and commitment to learn and practise during pregnancy. Ideally you'd want to start around 25 weeks into your pregnancy, but if you're a quick learner and put the time in, you may benefit from it later on. Hypnobirthing techniques can be used through any stage of labour and it is best to learn with a birth partner, although you can learn the techniques by yourself if you do not have one.

/ **TENS MACHINE**. Transcutaneous electrical nerve stimulation is often used in labour and involves electrodes, connected to a small handheld device, being placed on your back. These electrodes transmit small impulses to stimulate the nerves that run to the uterus and cervix. The idea is that these impulses block pain signals to the brain. There is not a huge amount of evidence that this approach has much of an effect in established labour, but TENS may be able to help you in the early stages. This can be used in conjunction with hypnobirthing, Entonox and opiates if you wish.

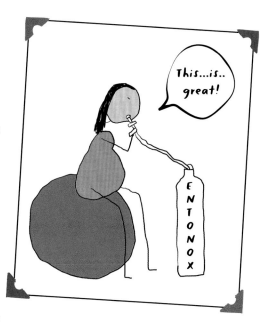

Pharmacological

/ **ENTONOX (GAS AND AIR)**. Entonox is a colourless, odourless gas made up of 50 per cent oxygen and 50 per cent nitrous oxide. It's also known as laughing gas, or gas and air, and is mainly used as a form of pain relief during established labour. It can help take the edge off pain rather than blocking it out completely, and you may also find that it makes you feel light-headed and giggly, like you've had a couple of glasses of wine! Entonox is usually available wherever you choose to give birth, including birth centres, home and hospitals.

In hospital, it is commonly available from a central supply in the wall so that it can be given to you 'on tap' whenever you need it. If you're in a hospital or a birth centre without a central supply, or if you're having a homebirth, your midwife can bring gas and air to you in portable cylinders. Entonox is administered through a mouthpiece in most hospitals and birth centres, although some use masks which may be a little more uncomfortable. You inhale on the Entonox continuously through a contraction, putting it down when the contraction is over. There are no known side-effects to the baby and it doesn't cross the placenta to the baby. If used excessively (puffing away even when there's not a contraction, or breathing on it too fast) it may cause nausea, vomiting or a feeling of being 'out of control'. It's not for everyone but it's definitely worth considering.

/ **OPIOIDS**. Opioids are sometimes used in labour if things become increasingly intense. Most hospitals offer them in the form of pethidine, meptid and/or diamorphine. These are injections, usually given in your buttocks, which make you feel drowsy. Opioids work by helping make you feel relaxed and less receptive to the pain of the contractions. You may also find that you become sleepy, nodding off in between contractions. Opioids do cross the placenta though, so shouldn't be given too close to the birth of the baby as it may affect their breathing. Opioids can also have an impact on the baby's ability to feed after birth.

Opioids can make you feel nauseous so an anti-sickness medication is often given at the same time as the opioid. They generally wear off after a few hours, so you may have multiple doses if you are in labour for a long time. Opioids can be combined with Entonox and are readily available in hospitals and most birth centres.

/ **EPIDURAL**. An epidural is a form of anaesthesia that delivers a full pain block when effective, but it does come with more risks than other forms of pain relief, as administering it requires an invasive procedure. It can be helpful for women who are having extremely long labours and are exhausted, and need the chance to rest before the birth. An epidural is a mixture of drugs, typically made up of a local anaesthetic and an opioid.

When you have an epidural, an area of skin is numbed on your lower back, then a thin catheter tube is passed through into what is called the epidural space. The drugs are pushed into this space, effectively numbing the area (blocking the pain signals sent up to your brain by your nerves). The tube remains in place throughout labour and can be topped up by the anaesthetist or controlled by you using a PCA (patient-controlled analgesia) device.

If you have an epidural it will be recommended that you don't eat or drink, other than sip water. This is because it is thought that having an epidural may increase the chances of you needing a caesarean. For a caesarean, having an empty stomach reduces the risk of lung aspiration should you need a general anaesthetic. There is still a lot of debate about whether epidurals actually increase the chance of having a caesarean. Some evidence suggests that they may prolong labour, and that they come with a higher chance of having a birth assisted with

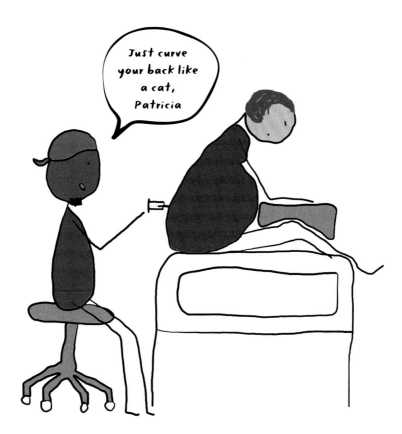

forceps. To keep you hydrated, a drip will be placed in a vein in your arm. Your blood pressure will be checked regularly as epidurals can cause it to drop, and your baby's heartbeat will also need to be continuously monitored.

You can opt for an epidural regardless of whether you have tried any of the other forms of pain management first, even if it wasn't in your plan to have one. Epidurals give complete pain relief in around 90 per cent of cases, and often the nerve block is heavy so you cannot feel your legs. This makes it difficult to move and mobilise. Going to the toilet may be tricky, so a catheter may be placed into your bladder to prevent it from becoming overly full. If

considering an epidural, it's worth asking for a 'low dose' or 'mobile' epidural. This lower-strength concoction allows for more movement of the limbs during labour.

You might experience itching and uneven patches of numbness around the body, and there are some less-common side effects that an anaesthetist will discuss with you thoroughly if you decide to have an epidural.

Epidurals are generally considered safe, but your care provider will discuss all the potential side effects with you beforehand so that you can make an informed choice. They are only given in hospitals as they require an anaesthetist to administer them.

Monitoring In Labour

During labour, you and your baby will be monitored to check your wellbeing.

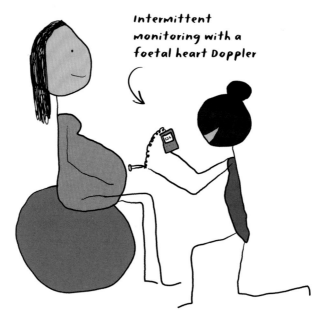

Intermittent monitoring with a foetal heart Doppler

Monitoring you

When you have an initial assessment in labour, the midwife will take a brief history from you and then carry out some observations. These will include measuring your blood pressure, pulse, respiratory rate, temperature and taking a urine sample. Doing this helps pick up any warning signs or indications of a potential problem such as an infection, blood clot or high blood pressure. You will also be asked about any vaginal loss, i.e. water, discharge or blood. You may or may not have noticed this in your underwear or during a trip to the toilet.

As labour progresses, monitoring will continue, usually with your pulse being checked every half an hour, and temperature plus blood pressure every four hours (or hourly if you're having an epidural). Your midwife will also make a note of how often you are contracting, how strong the contractions are, how often you are passing urine and if there is any vaginal loss, on a regular basis.

Monitoring your baby

The vast majority of babies sail through labour and the intensity of contractions safely with no problems. Occasionally, however, a baby may show signs of distress during labour, so listening to the baby's heartbeat is a part of labour care that is offered and recommended. By listening to the baby's heart tones, your care provider can detect any unusual rhythms.

Monitoring your baby's heartbeat during labour can be done in a number of ways. If you have enjoyed a straightforward pregnancy and have gone into labour spontaneously, with no concerns, intermittent monitoring with a handheld electrical Doppler or Pinard stethoscope can be used. In the UK, guidelines recommend that all women with uncomplicated pregnancies should be monitored intermittently every fifteen minutes once in established labour, checking both you and your baby's heart rates throughout and after a contraction. This allows you to mobilise freely and even go for a short walk around the unit or at home if you want. Evidence suggests that routine use of CTG monitoring (see below) in an uncomplicated pregnancy has no impact on improving perinatal outcomes. In other words, it's seldom necessary and in fact being able to move around in labour is likely to be more beneficial.

If the labour is deemed to be complex, or there are already other interventions in place (i.e. being induced with the used of synthetic oxytocin, having an epidural, or labouring with twins or multiples), continuous monitoring via a CTG (cardiotocograph) machine may be recommended and offered.

Continuous monitoring involves having two pads strapped to your abdomen. One records the baby's heart rate and the other your contractions. Over a period of time, usually at least twenty minutes, the recording is interpreted via a chart to see if baby is coping well. They look at the pattern of the baby's heart rate, and how it relates to the contractions.

Some reasons for continuous monitoring via CTG include:

- Induction of labour.
- Meconium-stained waters.
- Epidural.
- Bleeding during labour.
- Twin or multiple pregnancy.
- Preterm labour.
- Severe pre-eclampsia.
- IUGR (Intrauterine growth restriction).
- Abnormal foetal heart rate heard when listening intermittently with a Doppler.
- Reduced foetal movements.

If you have a complex pregnancy or labour and it's recommended you have continuous monitoring, you don't necessarily have to lie strapped on the bed. You can always ask if they have wireless telemetry monitors so that you can move around or, if not, sit on a birthing ball or chair next to the bed. This will help labour progress more easily and will most likely be more comfortable for you!

Occasionally it can become difficult to detect the baby's heart rate externally via an abdominal CTG, particularly if the pads that are attached to you keep slipping off or if the baby continuously moves. If there are concerns over the baby's wellbeing and continuous tracing of the heart is needed, a foetal scalp electrode may be suggested. A foetal scalp electrode is connected to the CTG machine at one end, and the other end is attached to the baby's head through the cervix via a hook which clips onto the baby's scalp.

You may want to discuss foetal monitoring with your care provider prior to having your baby if you are unsure which type will be recommended for you.

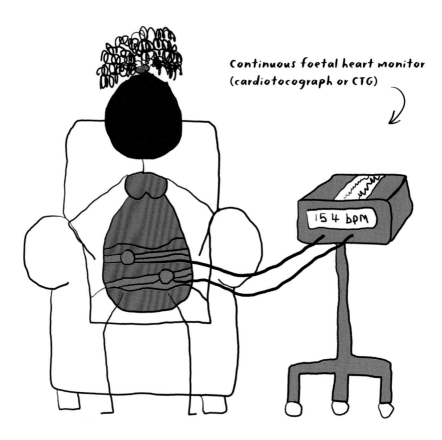

Continuous foetal heart monitor (cardiotocograph or CTG)

154 bpm

Assisted Birth:
ventouse or forceps

An assisted birth is one which happens with the help of an obstetric doctor using a medical instrument. There are two methods for this: ventouse (also known as suction/vacuum birth) or forceps.

There are a number of reasons why a ventouse or forceps birth might be performed. It could be that you are exhausted and are finding it difficult to push the baby out, or perhaps the baby's head is in a tricky position, making it difficult to be born, or maybe the baby is close to being born but there is concern for their wellbeing so a quick birth is indicated. Assisted births can only take place if the cervix is fully dilated and the baby is able to pass through.

Ventouse

A ventouse is a metal or silicone suction cup which is placed on the baby's head by the obstetrician. A vacuum is used to help guide the baby through and out of the birth canal while the mother pushes during contractions. The doctor will only attempt to guide baby down a few times before considering alternative methods of birth, most

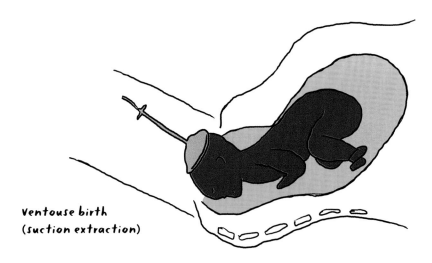

Ventouse birth
(suction extraction)

likely forceps or caesarean. After a ventouse birth, the baby will often have some swelling on the head, which will usually reduce within a day or so. Babies who are born via ventouse have a slightly increased chance of having jaundice in the first few days of life. This is something that the midwife will assess when visiting you in the days after the birth. Most cases of jaundice are mild and resolve themselves on their own. You can read more about jaundice on page 228.

Forceps

Forceps are basically like a big pair of tongs. They are designed to help turn the baby's head if they are in a non-optimal position for birth. Like the ventouse, forceps guide the baby down the birth canal as you push through each contraction. Forceps are more likely to require an episiotomy, as more space is needed in the vagina to use the forceps. You should receive a local anaesthetic before any cut is made.

If it is not possible to bring the baby out using forceps, the next step would be to consider caesarean birth. A baby who has been born via forceps may have forcep marks on their face, but these usually disappear within a few days of birth.

The Royal College of Obstetricians and Gynaecologists offers some useful guidance on things you can do to avoid an assisted birth. Remaining upright, or on your side, during labour and birth can help. Avoiding epidurals can also reduce the need for an assisted birth. If you do have an epidural, however, extra time should be given at the end of labour when you are fully dilated to allow the head to drop as low down into the birth canal as possible. This makes pushing your baby out much easier and helps prevent exhaustion.

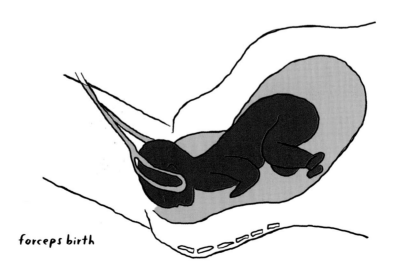

forceps birth

Caesarean Birth

Some women will give birth via caesarean (also known as c-section) and this can be planned or unplanned. If you have a caesarean planned, it's much easier to prepare for it. If you don't, it's always good to know what to expect just in case.

A caesarean is a surgical procedure whereby an incision is made in the lower abdomen to birth the baby. In most cases the cut is performed horizontally just at the bikini line. Occasionally, a vertical incision is made, but this is generally only performed in exceptional circumstances, for example with a preterm baby that is in a difficult position in the uterus.

Caesareans may be scheduled in for a variety of reasons. If you have had one previously, occasionally VBAC (vaginal birth after caesarean) isn't advised. This is often the case with women who have previously had a classical (vertical) incision rather than a lower horizontal one, or women who had a caesarean but are now pregnant with twins or a breech baby. Other reasons for a planned caesarean may include an unstable lie – baby could be lying across the uterus in a transverse position which would make vaginal birth difficult – or placenta praevia, when the placenta is too close to or covering the cervix.

Caesareans are major abdominal surgery and should not be taken lightly. Your experience and recovery will depend on many factors and everyone's experience is unique. If it has been suggested that you have a planned caesarean, do ask the reasons behind the suggestion and if you are unsure at all, make sure you do your research before making your own informed decision. Prior to a caesarean, a number of things will happen to ensure the procedure goes as smoothly as possible. If the caesarean is planned, the preparation will start at home. You may be asked to do a few things, including:

- Not to eat past midnight on the day prior to surgery.
- Shave your pubic hair just below the bikini line. (Some hospitals may ask that you wait until you're admitted for this.)
- To ensure you have no nail varnish or acrylic nails as well as no makeup.

This is so that the anaesthetist can check your nail bed and skin tone if required, to ensure adequate oxygenation. (Check with your hospital.)

- To take your prescribed antacid medication if given.

If you have an unplanned caesarean, you won't be able to avoid the fact that you may have eaten prior to surgery but don't worry, you will be given an antacid to prevent reflux if a general anaesthetic is required. Reflux under general anaesthetic is extremely rare these days, but the precaution is still in place in most hospitals. The nurses or midwives will shave your pubic hair for you, and they will ask you to remove jewellery if there is time.

In the event of either a planned or unplanned caesarean, there will be a consent form to sign and a review with the surgeon/anaesthetist who will discuss the reasons for – and risks of – the proposed surgery. In an emergency, this chat often occurs on the way to theatre.

What happens in the operating theatre?

The operating room can look daunting at first, with all the equipment and people, but when you get to know what everything's for, it won't seem too scary! Most operating rooms only allow one person to come and support you, as there's not much space in the room, and often women will have the father of the baby or their partner with them.

During the surgery, there are a number of other people there with you and – in the UK – these include:

- Surgeon (obstetric doctor) to perform the caesarean.
- Surgeon's assistant, often a more junior doctor.
- Anaesthetist, to ensure you don't feel a thing.
- ODP (operating department practitioner) to keep the theatre organised.
- Midwife to receive the baby and support the parent(s).
- Paediatrician in the case of an emergency caesarean or known concerns with the baby.
- Runner or maternity assistant to support the rest of the team.

Once you're in the operating room, the team's first task is to numb the lower half of your body. A spinal anaesthetic will usually be given if you haven't already got an epidural in place. If it's an emergency caesarean, your epidural may just be topped up. You will need a cannula in your hand or arm: access to your veins is important, for the anaesthetist to administer medications quickly as and when necessary. A catheter will be inserted into your bladder, as the anaesthetic will cause you to lose the ability to pee.

Once the anaesthetic is given, you will be laid down and after a few minutes the surgical team will test how effective the numbing anaesthetic is before they begin. This is usually done with a cold spray or by gently pinching your skin. Drapes are put over your body so that the only area visible is your abdomen. A screen is also put up so that you can't see the operation taking place! At this point, in order to remain calm and relaxed, it may be helpful to try focusing on hypnobirthing breathing techniques, or clearing your mind

66

Aside from mopping your brow with a cool cloth, ensuring you have plenty of water, or lending a hand to squeeze, a birth partner should be able to act as your advocate.

99

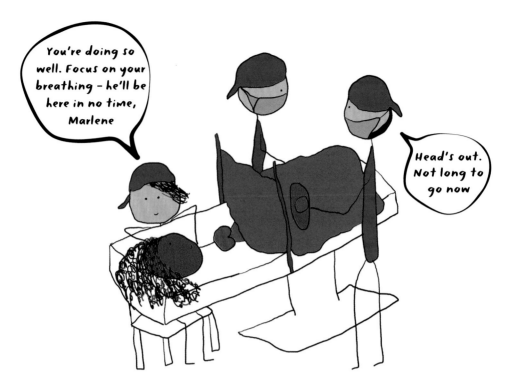

by visualising a happy, serene setting such as a beach or a waterfall. Chatting to your partner may also act as a distraction and give a sense of security. There may be lots of machines beeping but this is totally normal. Some operating rooms allow music to be played, so request this if it is something you would like during the birth.

Your birth partner should be able to sit close by at your head end. The anaesthetist is there to ensure that you are physically stable throughout the operation. Use them to communicate your concerns if you feel unwell at any stage. The midwife or assistant will shave any pubic hair that is over the bikini line to make the surgery easier and cleaner, and to reduce the chance of ingrowing hairs afterwards. Your abdomen will be cleaned with an antibacterial wash (often orange in colour) to reduce the risk of infection.

Once the surgery begins, the baby is often out in under ten minutes. You will remain in the operating room for another forty-five minutes to one hour, while the surgeons finish suturing your wound and check all is well with you. When the baby is born, the umbilical cord is cut – you can request optimal cord clamping (see page 113) so long as baby doesn't need immediate resuscitation or any other urgent care. Once the cord is cut, your baby will be passed to you. Holding your baby after a caesarean is a great way to get the natural oxytocin hormones flowing to help with keeping your womb contracted, bonding and breastfeeding. If the baby needs immediate support at birth, they will be taken to a special cot that has lights, heating and all the equipment to support them. Once they are stable, they will be brought over to you. You may be given an analgesic in the form of a suppository (a small meltable tablet that is inserted into the rectum), which will help when the spinal or epidural wears off. You will also be given other drugs including an oxytocic to contract your womb, along with fluids through your cannula to keep you hydrated.

When will they perform the operation?

Most hospitals categorise how soon a caesarean should be performed with a grading system:

- **Category 4** — The operation will take place at a time that suits you and the caesarean team.
- **Category 3** — The baby needs to be born early but there is no immediate risk to you or your baby.
- **Category 2** — There are problems affecting the health of you and/or baby but they are not immediately life-threatening.
- **Category 1** — Immediate threat to the life of you or baby.

Category 3 and 4 caesareans are usually planned in advance but category 1 caesareans should take place within half an hour of the decision being made, and a little later for category 2. When I had a caesarean birth for my twins at 34 weeks' gestation, I went in for a routine ultrasound which showed that one of the twins' placentas was not functioning properly. They had been monitoring his growth over the previous few weeks. A decision was made to perform a category 2 caesarean that day and I gave birth a few hours later.

What happens after surgery?

When the surgery is complete, you should be wheeled on the bed to a recovery area where you will be closely monitored by a midwife or nurse. During this time you should be able to have skin-to-skin contact with your baby and offer them their first feed. If breastfeeding, many women find it easier to lie on their side after the surgery. If you find this tricky, you can try the classic cradle hold, but keep a pillow on your lap as the pressure of the baby can cause discomfort on your wound. You may feel nauseous, groggy, shaky and/or itchy after surgery – this is often a result of the medications given during the operation but is only temporary. Food and drink is not usually offered straight away, as there is an increased risk of you vomiting due to the medication. You will probably get to drink after half to one hour, and eat a little after that. In the UK, women are taken to the postnatal ward after the initial recovery period. You may stay in hospital anywhere between 1 and 3 days, or longer if there are issues (such as infection) that need addressing before you return home.

All this information may seem overwhelming now but remember there will always be someone to ask for help, support and advice in the hospital should you need it during or after a caesarean.

VBAC – Vaginal Birth After Caesarean

'Once a caesarean, always a caesarean.' That used to be a phrase that was spoken far too often many years ago.

It was always assumed that if you had a caesarean, any subsequent children would also need to be born this way. Things have changed drastically and now, in the UK, most people who have had one straightforward caesarean are encouraged to plan for a VBAC if that's their preference and they are enjoying an otherwise uncomplicated pregnancy. The discussion around how a subsequent baby is born after a caesarean is ultimately one that occurs in pregnancy between you and your care provider.

The main concern for someone who attempts a vaginal birth after caesarean is uterine scar rupture. A rupture is a tear in the uterine wall which is an emergency situation that can cause complications for both mother and baby. During a caesarean, several layers of skin and flesh are cut to get to the baby. The uterus is left with a scar which in most cases heals well with no issue. Uterine rupture after caesarean happens rarely, in around 0.5 per cent of labours in the UK, which is 1 in 200. VBAC is recommended by the Royal College of Obstetricians and Gynaecologists in otherwise uncomplicated situations and ideally there should be at least 18 months between births. A VBAC wouldn't be advised if you previously had a classical caesarean incision (vertical as opposed to horizontal).

When planning a VBAC, it's generally recommended you give birth in a hospital. Birth centres are unlikely to accept those who have previously had a caesarean because they do not have the facilities available should a repeat caesarean be indicated. If you are keen on giving birth in a birth centre, however, you can always have a discussion with the team to see if it's a possibility. Some birth centres are attached to labour wards so it would be an easy transfer should assistance be required.

Some people who are hoping for a VBAC choose to give birth at home. If a homebirth is something you are hoping for, discuss it with your midwife so you can weigh up all of the risks and benefits to help you make an informed decision.

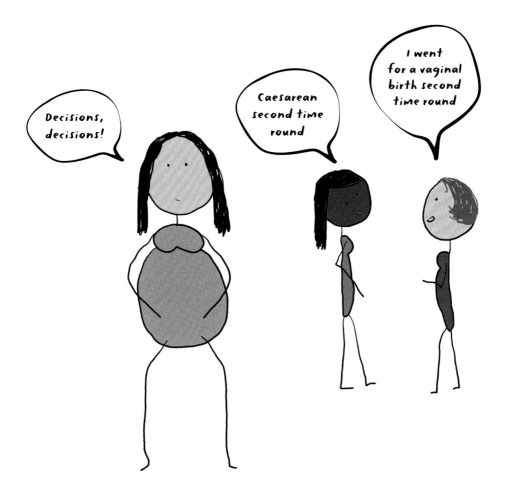

Had more than one previous caesarean?

There is a lot of discussion among experts around having a VBAC if there have been two previous caesareans. Studies have found that there were actually no significant differences in risk of uterine rupture if there have been one or two previous caesareans. Each situation is individual, however, and if you have had more than one caesarean in the past, your current birth should be discussed with your doctor and midwife.

The success rate for VBACs in the UK currently sits at around 75 per cent. It's as high as 85–90 per cent for women who had also previously had a vaginal birth as well as a caesarean, which is pretty great really. More information and stats on VBAC can be found at *rcog.org.uk*.

Complications During Birth

While most births are relatively straightforward, occasionally there can be unforeseen complications. Although experiencing any of these issues is unlikely, it can help to have an understanding of them.

Breech

Most babies are born head first – otherwise known as cephalic presentation. Although this is the most common and ideal position, sometimes a baby presents bottom or feet first, with their head at the top end of the uterus. This is known as breech and it makes vaginal birth a little trickier.

There are a few different variations of breech – complete, footling and frank (see page 73). Vaginal birth of a breech baby needs to be facilitated by a skilled midwife or doctor who can manage and support the birth in the appropriate way.

If your baby is in a breech position at 36 weeks, you may be offered an external cephalic version (ECV). This is when an obstetrician tries to turn the baby into a head-down position by applying pressure on your abdomen. It can be a bit uncomfortable, but around 50 per cent of breech babies can be turned using ECV. When an ECV has taken place, you will be monitored closely for a while afterwards to ensure all is well with the baby. As with many interventions, there are risks associated with an ECV. About 1 in 200 babies in the UK will require delivery by caesarean straight after an ECV due to complications (such as bleeding from the placenta, which may cause foetal distress). Sometimes a baby may also flip back into the breech position, and in this situation you will need to decide whether to go ahead and give birth vaginally or plan a caesarean.

Some women want to explore the possibility of having a breech vaginal birth rather than having an ECV or caesarean. This can be discussed with the obstetrician: they should be able to provide you with all of the information and stats required to help you make an informed decision.

Some scenarios where a breech vaginal birth would not be recommended include:

- Having a low-lying placenta.
- If the baby's head is tilted too far back, making the birth of the head difficult.
- If the baby is a 'footling breech' – feet first rather that bum first.
- If you have pre-eclampsia.
- You may have your own reasons for a planned caesarean being the best option.

There are also some things that you can try yourself, to encourage baby to turn. Moxibustion is a form of reflexology that is thought to help turn a baby into a head-down position. Several studies support the theory of moxibustion and there are many reflexologists who offer the treatment. Adopting different positions such as the forward-leaning inversion may also help. Ask your care provider if they support you trying these methods first, before you go ahead.

Sometimes a breech baby isn't diagnosed until a person is in labour. A discussion about the birth with your care provider will take place at the time, to decide the best mode of birth for you and your baby.

Cord prolapse

Sometimes, when a person's waters have broken, it's possible for the umbilical cord to slip past the baby's head and out into the vagina through the cervix (as the baby's head then sits on top of the cord it can compress it, cutting off the oxygen supply). This is known as a cord prolapse and will require urgent attention to bring the baby into the world as quickly as possible.

Cord prolapse is a risk if your waters break prematurely and the baby's head is still high above the pelvis, or if the baby is breech or in an unstable position such as lying transverse across the uterus. Ideally, the baby's head should be compressed against the cervix, preventing anything from getting past it, other than the odd trickle of amniotic fluid. When the head is deeply engaged in the pelvis, it is low down, blocking the cord from being able to pass through.

If you are already in stage two of labour and birth is imminent, a vaginal birth might be the quickest way for baby to be born. If you are not in labour, or the cervix isn't fully dilated, then the safest way would be to perform a caesarean. If you are not in hospital and part of the cord comes out when your waters break, get on your knees, bum in the air and face down, to relieve pressure from baby's head on the cord and stay like that. Call the emergency services to transport you to hospital ASAP. Luckily this is a rare occurrence, but it does happen in 0.1–0.6 per cent of births in the UK.

Shoulder dystocia

Shoulder dystocia is another rare event that can happen in 0.5–0.7 per cent of vaginal births. It occurs during the second stage of labour, when the head has been born. Usually the body follows straight after, but with a shoulder dystocia, one of the shoulders becomes stuck behind the mother's pelvic bone.

If a shoulder dystocia is suspected during the birth, the midwife will summon assistance and will encourage you to bring your knees right up towards your chest: usually that is enough to dislodge the shoulder but, if not, some pressure may be applied to your abdomen and you may be encouraged to roll onto all-fours. Occasionally, when these things don't work, the midwife or doctor may need to manually free the shoulder to expedite the birth. In the vast majority of cases, the baby will be born quickly and safely after this help.

It is difficult for clinicians to predict shoulder dystocia but there are thought to be some risk factors, including: macrosomia (baby weight over 4kg), twins or multiples and gestational diabetes. It is important to note, however, that despite these stats, most big babies are born vaginally without shoulder dystocia and, in fact, most babies born with shoulder dystocia are born with a normal weight!

Postpartum haemorrhage (PPH)

It's absolutely normal to lose blood from the vagina after having your baby, regardless of whether it's a caesarean or vaginal birth.

Normal blood loss is below 500ml. If blood loss is 500ml–1 litre, it's considered a minor PPH (higher than usual blood loss, but unlikely to cause any significant harm). If it's over 1 litre, it's considered serious. Most PPHs happen immediately after the birth and many are due to the uterus not contracting down straight away and constricting the blood vessels at the site where the placenta was attached. This can happen if there are bits of the placenta or membrane sac that weren't expelled. During the birth, if the bladder is full, that can also make it difficult for the uterus to contract down properly. In this instance, a catheter may be used to empty the bladder. Sometimes PPH is caused by perineal/vaginal tears that cut through a blood vessel.

If your doctor or midwife suspects a PPH after birth, they will check to make sure the placenta is completely out and rub the fundus (top of your uterus) from the outside to stimulate it to contract. If the bleeding continues, further steps are taken, usually in the form of drugs that will help to control it.

Several factors may increase your risk of having a PPH, including:

- Placenta praevia.
- Carrying twins or multiples.
- Having high blood pressure.
- Carrying a large baby.
- Induction of labour.
- Retained placenta.
- Blood-clotting issues or taking blood-thinning drugs in labour.
- Fibroids.
- Having an assisted birth or caesarean.

A PPH can happen any time within a couple of months of giving birth. It's more likely, however, in the first twenty-four hours. A PPH that occurs after the first twenty-four hours is called a secondary PPH.

Keep an eye on your postnatal blood loss by checking how often you are changing pads. If you are soaking through more than one an hour then you need to inform your care provider. You may notice blood clots in the first few days but let your care provider know if they are bigger than the size of a plum.

If you feel unwell, dizzy or nauseous then, again, make sure you let your care provider know.

Obstructed labour

Cephalopelvic disproportion (CPD) is a condition in which the baby's head is unable to pass through the pelvis as it is larger than the pelvis inlet. Many studies have confirmed that this condition is often over-diagnosed, and found that women who have had a caesarean due to this diagnosis have often gone on to give birth vaginally with a similar or bigger-sized baby.

Studies into true CPD have suggested that only 10 per cent of babies born to women diagnosed with CPD are macrosomic (large babies over 4kg). It's also thought that many true cases of CPD occur with people who have pelvic anomalies or injuries.

Carrying a large baby does not mean that you will not be able to birth them vaginally. Often a diagnosis of CPD is given when labour is slow or stalls. It's more likely to be an issue with the position of the baby's head rather than the size. True cephalopelvic disproportion can only be diagnosed by measuring the size and shape of the pelvis and the baby's head with a scanner, something that is unlikely to occur in the middle of labour!

The pelvis has ligaments that hold it together to allow it to stretch as the baby is descending. The skull is also soft, allowing it to 'mould' through the birth canal. Being active in labour, and moving into different positions if it starts to slow, can be a good way of helping the head descend.

So, what does all this mean, Marley? It means that just because you're pregnant with a possibly larger-than-average baby, that doesn't mean you won't be able to give birth vaginally. It also means that a longer labour is more likely to be a positional or emotional thing, as opposed to your pelvis being too small.

Preterm birth

Babies need around 40 weeks to fully grow and develop, but occasionally, a little one may decide to put in an appearance much earlier than this. When a baby is born before 37 weeks of pregnancy, it is considered to be a preterm or premature birth. In the UK, this affects around 7 per cent of births annually, which equates to around 60,000 premature babies.

It's important to note that not all of these premature babies will be born extremely early – many will be just a few days shy of the 37-week mark, and most of those will do very well.

According to research carried out by the pregnancy and birth charity Tommy's:

- 5 per cent of preterm births are extremely premature (before 28 weeks' gestation).
- 11 per cent are very preterm (28–32 weeks' gestation).
- 85 per cent are moderately preterm (32–37 weeks' gestation).

The outcome for the baby will largely depend on how long they were in the womb for; a baby born at 34 weeks is likely to do better than a baby born at 27 weeks. Neonatal intensive care units (NICU) are fantastic at caring for babies born early when all efforts to prevent a preterm birth have not worked. The earlier a baby is born, the longer they will usually spend in hospital as they gain weight, stabilise their breathing and learn to feed.

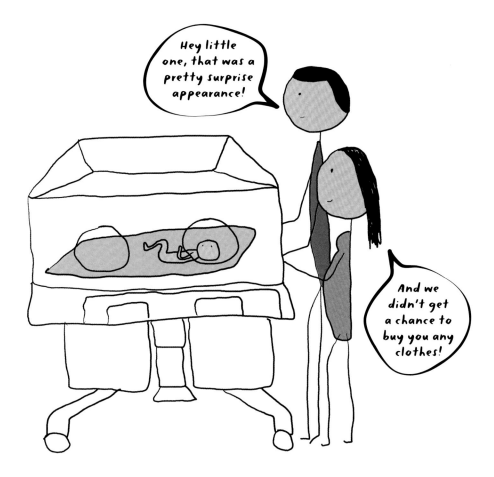

There are several factors that make preterm birth more likely, including:

- Drug and alcohol abuse.
- Untreated UTIs.
- Heavy smoking.
- Previous preterm birth.
- Carrying twins or multiples.
- Cervical or uterine issues.
- Physical trauma, such as a car accident.
- Pre-eclampsia.

Sometimes preterm births just occur with no known cause. If you are less than 37 weeks' pregnant and think you may be in labour, it's important to contact your care provider as soon as possible. If you are in labour, the next steps will depend on your gestation and how far into labour you are. With preterm babies, each day in the womb counts, so the goal would be to keep you pregnant for as long as possible, providing it's safe to do so. If labour cannot be stopped, you may be given steroids to help strengthen the baby's lungs when they are born.

Birth Partners
And Doulas

Having a support person/people during your birth providing practical help and advocacy can really make a difference to your entire experience. This section explores the roles of both birth partners and professional birth support (doulas).

Birth partners

Birth partners have a huge role to play during labour and birth and can be invaluable when it comes to providing support and advocacy when things can become intense. A good place to start is by involving your birth partner with creating your birth preferences plan.

Although ultimately your birth preferences are centred around your needs and wishes, it is good for your partner to get involved with supporting the decision-making process. Labour and birth can make you feel extremely vulnerable and not always able to speak up and ask questions if you need to. So, aside from the physical aspect i.e. mopping your brow with a cool cloth and ensuring you have plenty of water, or lending a hand to squeeze, a birth partner should be able to act as your advocate. Sometimes women need someone to help explain to health professionals what they want, especially if they are in the throes of labour!

In early labour, having someone to talk to and distract you is also something that a birth partner can do, as well as offer words of encouragement when labour becomes more intense.

No matter who your birth partner is – the baby's father, your mum, partner, friend, sister, etc. – their role involves more than simply watching the baby enter the world. It can be a long and tiring process for both of you, but there are plenty of things that they can do to help!

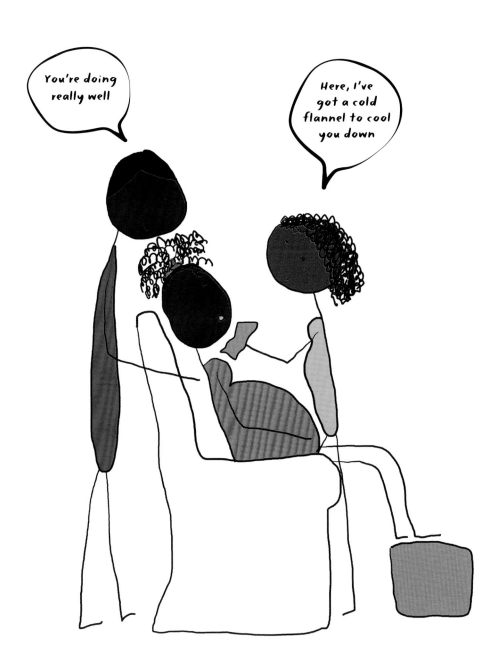

Here are a few tips for your birth partner to read:

- Create a calm environment: low lights, music etc.
- Offer massage, a hug, or to hold her hand. If she declines, don't worry!
- Offer her water or food if she is able to eat. Keep a cool towel for her brow if she becomes too warm.
- Offer comforts such as lavender oil, pillows or blankets from home.
- During transitional labour, try to keep her calm and focused by speaking gently and giving her positive affirmations, noting how well she is doing.

Being present throughout labour and birth can also be overwhelming for the birth partner. Birth partners should make sure they keep topped up with fluids and snacks so that they have maximum energy to offer their support to their partners.

Doulas

A doula is a person who provides physical, practical, emotional and informational support to you and your partner during pregnancy, childbirth and the postnatal period. A doula's role and agenda are solely linked to your wishes and their responsibility is to you – not to the hospital, midwife or doctor. A birth doula supports you during pregnancy, labour and birth and a postnatal doula offers hands-on support in your home as you adjust to parenthood.

/ BIRTH DOULA

Having a professional who is experienced in supporting people through labour and birth and understands the process, as well as one that knows you and your wishes, can really make a difference to your experience. Most birth doulas will start their support at your home during pregnancy and the early stages of labour, and if you're planning to give birth in hospital, transfer with you when the time comes. Some of the things a birth doula can offer during labour and birth include:

- Continuity of support.
- Attention to physical comfort through techniques such as touch and massage.
- Offering reassurance, encouragement, praise and nurturing.
- Explanations of procedures and information about what's happening in labour.
- Help with facilitating communication between you and the hospital staff.
- Support for your birth partner.
- Helping you adjust into various positions to help labour progress.
- Assistance with breastfeeding.

Studies have shown that continuous support from doulas during childbirth may result in:

- An increased likelihood of a spontaneous vaginal birth.
- A lower rate of medicated analgesia use.
- A lower chance of having a caesarean.
- A reduced length of labour.
- A higher rate of positive birth experiences.

/ POSTNATAL DOULA

Some of the things a postnatal doula can offer during the postnatal period:

- Routine newborn care, guidance for the parents in bathing, calming techniques, sleeping patterns and newborn development.
- Breastfeeding and/or formula feeding support.
- Household tasks including laundry, light housekeeping, grocery shopping and meal preparation.
- Care of older siblings.
- Accompany you and your baby to any appointments or shopping trips.
- Running errands.

Studies have shown that having a postnatal doula may result in:

- Greater breastfeeding success.
- Greater self-confidence.
- Less postnatal depression.

A doula is not a medical professional and doesn't provide medical advice, nor would they attempt to try and change the clinical recommendations of a midwife or an obstetrician – only you and your partner can do that. They can, however, offer evidence-based information and support based on their knowledge and experience, acting as an advocate, ensuring you understand your options so that you can make informed choices about your care.

To find out more about doulas and to find one in your area, visit *thedoulaassociation.org*.

For more research, visit *evidencebasedbirth.com/the-evidence-for-doulas*.

What Should I Pack In My Birth Bag?

This is the million-dollar question! There are so many different suggestions for what should be in a birth bag, many of which come from mothers themselves, so they can all be different and it can get pretty confusing. A birth bag is a collection of items to take with you to the hospital or birth centre (if that's where you're planning to give birth).

I have put together a simple birth-bag list for you, baby and your birth partner, which includes essentials and optional extras. If you are planning a homebirth, you might want to have this prepared in the event of a transfer to hospital. Keep reading to find a list of additional essentials for homebirth too!

Baby

Clothing

- Scratch mittens x 2
- Hats x 3
- Short-sleeved bodysuits x 6 (3 x newborn and 3 x 0–3 months)
- Long-sleeved onesies with closed feet x 6 (3 x newborn and 3 x 0–3 months)
- Nappies x 1 pack
- Cotton-wool balls or water-based wipes
- Outfit for going home – a onesie and vest if the weather is warm, or layer up with an additional cardigan if cold

Other

- Blankets x 2
- Muslin squares

Optional extras

- Baby hairbrush
- Nail cutters
- Harvested colostrum – must be named and dated, ready to go straight into the hospital fridge

You

Clothing

- Comfortable outfit for labour – nightgown/oversized T-shirt fine
- Nightgown/pyjamas x 2
- Dressing gown
- Slippers
- Socks x 4
- High-rise or disposable underwear x 6
- Comfortable outfit for day/to go home. Tracksuit or loose-fitting dress
- Nursing bras x 3

Accessories and cosmetics

- Hairbrush
- Toothbrush
- Toothpaste
- Flannel
- Body/face wash
- Deodorant
- Nipple cream
- Breast pads – you probably won't need these straight away
- Large towel
- Maternity pads x 1 pack
- Lip balm
- Moisturising cream
- Hair ties

Food and drink

- Refillable water bottle
- Snacks for labour – fruit, nuts, crackers, biscuits
- Energy drink
- Bottle of squash

Comfort and planning

- Pillow, ideally a nursing one
- Extra blanket if it's cold
- Birth preferences document

Gadgets

- Phone/camera
- Charger

Optional extras

- Music playlist/hypnobirthing MP3s (if enrolled on a course)
- Speakers (for music)
- TENS machine for pain management
- Fan
- Spray bottle for water
- Aromatherapy oils
- Birthing ball (if the facility doesn't have one)
- Swimwear/bikini top for water birth if you want!
- Straws, especially if you're planning a caesarean. You may find it uncomfortable to sit upright afterwards to drink, so these will come in handy.

Birth partner

- **Money**
  Plenty of loose change for the car park.

- **A small blanket**
  You may find yourself getting cold if the labour is overnight.

- **Comfortable shoes**
  There's nothing worse than pacing the corridor with your partner while wearing shoes that hurt your feet.

- **Toothbrush, toothpaste and deodorant**
  If it's a long day/night, you may want to freshen up.

- **Your own pillow**
  If you manage to catch a few minutes' rest between supporting your partner, a pillow many be useful.

- **A change of clothes**
  If you're at hospital for a long time, with no chance of a shower, clean clothes will help you feel that bit fresher. You may want to bring some shorts if it's hot, and extra clothing if it's cold.

- **Snacks and drinks**
  Your hospital or birth centre will likely have refreshments available, but it's a good idea to have what you need to hand – that way you won't need to leave your partner. The last thing you want is to end up hungry and dehydrated!

- **Swimwear**
  If your partner is planning a water birth you may want to get in the pool too to support her and be close when the baby is born.

- **Glasses, if you're a contact-lens wearer**
  Glasses will probably be more comfortable and will save you from having to change contacts.

- **Smartphone, digital camera or camcorder**
  You may want to capture pictures or videos of the birth or afterwards. Don't forget the chargers too!

What To Prepare For A Homebirth

If you have decided to have your baby at home, you may be wondering what you need to prepare. The first thing you should do is look at the lists on the previous pages and have a bag ready by the door in the unlikely event that you'll require a transfer to hospital.

Your midwife/midwives will bring all the medical kit that is required for the birth. If you are arranging a homebirth with your midwife, they should meet you at some point to discuss what will happen. They will also go over what you will need for the big day. In the meantime, though, here is a basic list that you may find useful:

- Maternity notes/birth preferences.
- Blankets and clean towels.
- Large plastic sheets to protect the carpets/sofa in the area where you are planning to give birth.
- Desk lamp with a bright bulb, so that the midwife can check your vagina and perineum after the birth.
- Bucket, just in case you vomit during labour.
- Several bin bags for rubbish.
- Any medication you take – keep this close to hand.
- Calming items for your environment, e.g. aromatherapy oils, candles, massage oil, music playlist.
- Birthing/yoga ball.
- Pool, if you intend to have a water birth. Set it up around a week before your due date and keep it covered until you are in labour and ready to fill it.
- Maternity pads.
- A comfortable outfit for birthing if you want to be covered.
- Snacks to keep you going.
- Tea/coffee for the midwives!

If you have pets, ensure there is a safe area in your home for them to stay while the midwives are with you during active labour.

All birth-related waste such as the placenta will be taken by the midwives to dispose of, unless you would like to keep it.

The Fourth Trimester

Trimester

& Postnatal Recovery

In This Chapter

Let's now explore what to expect after you have had your baby.

It's taken months to get to this point and now a brand new adventure awaits!

The fourth trimester, or postnatal (postpartum) stage, refers to the first 3-6 months after a baby is born, and the adjustments they make as they navigate their way through a new world of noise, bright lights, frequent changes of temperature and regular feelings of needing to eat. These are all things that they are experiencing for the first time, so it can be overwhelming for them. Meanwhile, you are recovering from the pregnancy and birth, both physically and emotionally. This chapter will help you to understand what to expect, along with tips on how to make the early days more manageable.

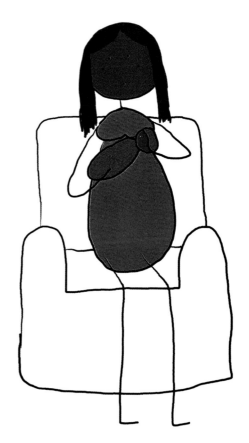

Skin To Skin And The 'Golden Hour'

Mothers and babies have an emotional and physiological need to be together at the moment of birth and during the hours and days that follow.

Care givers will always recommend immediate, uninterrupted skin-to-skin contact after vaginal birth, and during and after caesarean surgery if possible, regardless of how baby will be fed. As soon as your baby is born, it's likely your instinct will guide you to reach down and hold them. You will probably notice that after they cry initially, once they're lying on your chest with a towel laid over them, they slowly start to settle down again. This is probably because they can hear your heart beat and feel your warmth, which makes them begin to feel more relaxed.

Skin-to-skin contact provides a variety of health benefits and not just at birth. It can reduce both yours and baby's stress levels, helps to regulate the baby's body temperature, promotes oxytocin production and can slow down bleeding in mum as a result. It also increases the chances of successful breastfeeding.

Ideally, this special time should last for at least an hour: this period is referred to as the 'golden hour'. If you are planning on breastfeeding, skin to skin should help to initiate the process.

If, due to unforeseen circumstances, the golden hour doesn't happen (i.e. due to baby needing neonatal intensive care unit (NICU) support) don't worry too much: skin to skin can resume at a time when both you and baby are stable and it's safe to do so.

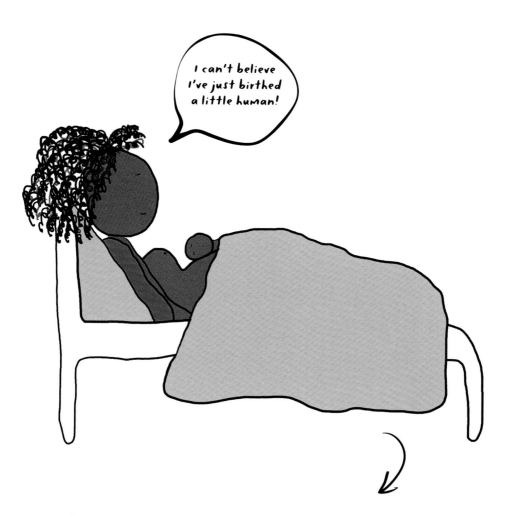

When babies are born, routine procedures like weighing and examinations can generally wait until you and your baby have had that special bonding time.

Newborn Examinations

Within minutes of a baby being born, the midwife will have assessed them using what's called an APGAR score. This tool is used to gauge your baby's wellbeing at one minute and five minutes after birth.

The APGAR score is also sometimes recorded at ten minutes, if necessary. This assessment can be done visually while baby is in your arms – there is no need to remove baby from you unless they appear to be unwell. So, here is what the APGAR score is actually looking at:

- *Appearance* (skin colour).
- *Pulse* (heart rate).
- *Grimace response* (reflexes, facial movements).
- *Activity* (muscle tone).
- *Respiration* (breathing rate).

Each factor is given a maximum of two points. For example, if a baby's skin colour appears normal, they will get a score of 2. If it's normal except the hands and feet, it would be 1. Once the APGAR assessment is complete, there should be a maximum of 10 points. It gives the care provider an idea of the baby's condition and whether they may need any intervention, respiratory assistance or observation.

Most babies' APGAR scores are around 8/9 at one minute and then 10 at five minutes. After the initial APGAR and period of skin-to-skin contact, a more thorough examination of the baby is done. Sometimes this can be carried out with baby still lying with you; if not, it should still be performed in the same room with you and your birth partner able to watch. The midwife will take your baby's temperature, record their respiratory rate and heart rate, check their head, face and mouth, torso, limbs, extremities, skin and genitals for any anomalies. The baby will also be weighed. It's a good idea at this stage to take a photograph of baby on the scales: it's a great keepsake and also avoids any confusion over the birth weight later on when you are at home!

APGAR score

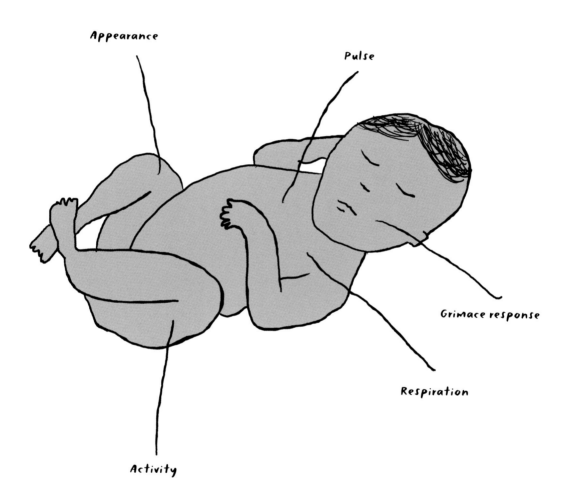

Appearance

Pulse

Grimace response

Respiration

Activity

Support In Hospital Or A Birth Centre

Shortly after you give birth, have had your golden time and have been supported in feeding your baby, it will be time to transfer you to the postnatal ward.

Postnatal wards have bay areas that are usually made up of four to eight beds that are occupied by different women. Each bed will have a curtain to ensure privacy and the chance to rest undisturbed, but being in an environment with other new mums may be an ideal opportunity to have a chat if you fancy it! If you would rather have a private room, you will have to request one once you have given birth. In NHS hospitals, these rooms are paid for on a first-come-first-served basis and will sometimes include a bathroom or shower. The care and food you receive will be exactly the same as if you were in one of the bay areas. Visiting hours will also be the same.

Before leaving the birthing ward, your midwife will assist you to the shower or, if you are unable to leave your bed due to an epidural/caesarean, will help to wash you in bed so that you are feeling a little more comfortable. You should be able to eat something light, too, before you are transferred to the postnatal ward.

When you arrive at the postnatal ward, it's good to find out where things are, such as the toilets and bathroom, whether breakfast is brought to you or if there is an area where you can make it yourself, where the water machine is and where the midwife station is. If you aren't mobile immediately, don't worry. You will have a call bell by your bed to press when you need assistance with things. You will have food brought to you and there's no reason why someone can't bring some food from home, too!

If you have decided to breastfeed, there should be support on the ward twenty-four hours a day from midwives, midwifery assistants and infant feeding specialists. The infant feeding team often work office hours, but there should always be someone around to help you with establishing and maintaining breastfeeding. If you decide to formula feed, find out where the preparation area is so that you can prepare milk safely.

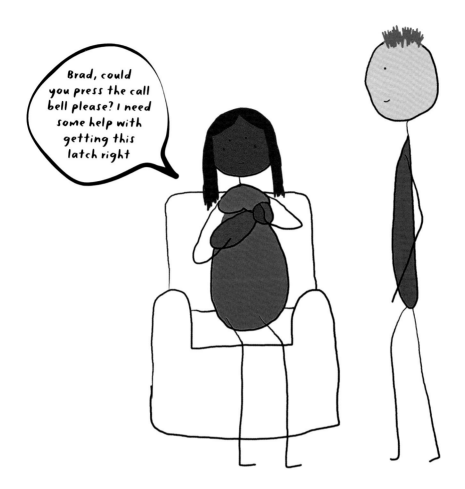

The length of time you stay in hospital or the birth centre largely depends on the type of birth you've had, and how well you and your baby are. Many first-time mothers will stay in overnight after having their baby. After a caesarean, this can be extended by a few days. Some find the extra time helps them gain confidence in looking after their baby, others like to go home sooner. As long as both you and your baby are okay and baby is feeding well, you have the option of heading off home six hours after the birth.

Before being discharged, a midwife will sit with you and give you information on what happens next – postnatal visits and appointments, health-visitor contact, where to register the birth, emergency contact numbers for the hospital, and more. When you are discharged home, be sure you have the correct car seat to carry your baby in. The regulations surrounding i-size car seats (car seats which meet European standards) can be found at *childcarseats.org.uk*. Ideally, someone should collect you and drive you and your baby home, whether that be a partner, family member, friend or taxi driver.

Afterpains

Afterpains can come as a bit of a shock to new mums, especially if you've never heard of them before. After giving birth, you will likely have experienced a sense of relief as your labour contractions ceased. Your uterus now, however, has the task of involuting (reducing in size).

Afterpains typically start a while after the birth, when you have had time to meet and bond with your baby, had something to eat and showered (or bed wash if you have had a caesarean), and generally caught your breath.

Afterpains often emerge when new mums start breastfeeding, as the feeding releases oxytocin, which tells your uterus to start contracting. Suddenly, you may begin to notice period-like cramps. Although it may feel pretty uncomfortable, it's usually nothing to be concerned about, just the uterus working towards getting back into its pre-pregnancy state. You may also notice that when the cramps occur, the bleeding becomes heavier as the uterus works to expel as much as possible.

You'll be pleased to know that not everyone notices these contractions after birth, especially first-time mothers. They tend to be something experienced more by women who have had at least one birth. With the more severe cases, it can feel like you are in early labour again! Hot water bottles and mild painkillers can help a lot.

Afterpains tend to last for at least twenty-four hours (I experienced them for a few days with the birth of my fifth baby), but if you do experience afterpains, be assured they are short lived: all the cramping will soon be overshadowed by the irresistible scent of your new baby and a flurry of snuggles.

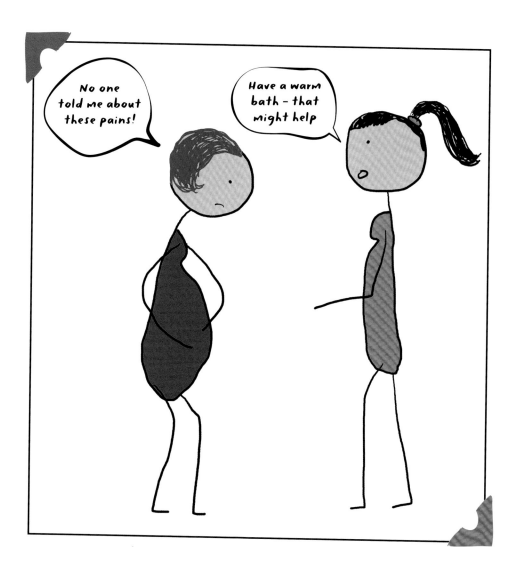

Going Home:
what to expect during your first night

Going home after having a baby, especially your first, can be incredibly nerve-racking. Having the responsibility of a newborn baby while trying to recover from giving birth can be daunting and particularly hard, more so if you don't have much in the way of support.

You may have been feeling euphoric in the hospital or birth centre, during the early hours after the birth, only to arrive home and feel the energy turn into tiredness. You will probably feel like doing nothing but resting and snuggling close to your baby. Babies tend to sleep quite a bit for the first twenty-four to forty-eight hours of their lives, which can lead you into a false sense of security about their sleep patterns. You may find that when you get home, they suddenly wake up and find their voice!

I suggest preparing for this moment while you are still pregnant, if you can (see pages 88–89).

When you get home, set up a spot on the sofa or bed. Keep a basket or box close by that contains a bottle of water, snacks, the remote control, a phone charger, nappies, medications, muslin/burp cloths and any other essentials that will prevent you from having to move around too much.

Although it might sound like a little bit of a cliché, try and catch a few minutes' sleep when your baby does, if you can. Your baby won't develop a sleeping pattern for some time, and this technique should help you feel less tired in the early days. If you have a partner to support you, assign them the washing and cleaning duties. Your focus should initially be on recovery and bonding. You may find it feels strange at home on the first night, but it won't be long before you adjust and settle into parenthood.

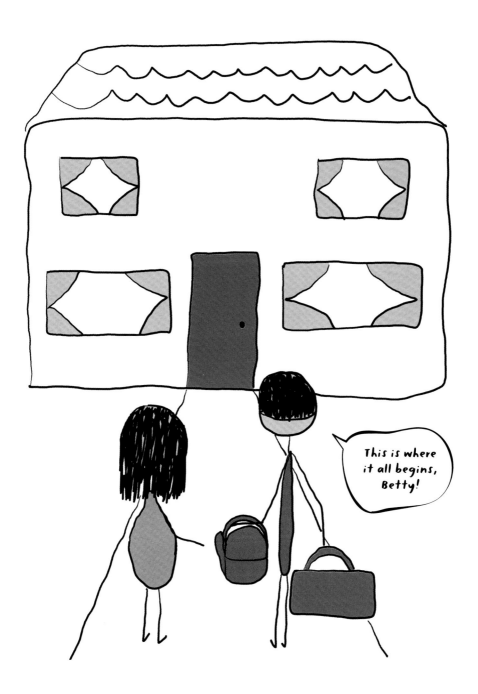

What The Fourth Trimester Means For Babies

Dr Harvey Karp, a renowned paediatrician, was credited for the popularity of the phrase 'the fourth trimester'. He suggests that even full-term babies are born 'too soon', and encourages parents to think of their babies as 'foetuses outside the womb' for the first 3–6 months of their lives. This might sound like a bizarre concept, but it actually makes sense when you think about it.

After spending many months in the uterus, not feeling hungry, being warm, secure and having every need met, suddenly your baby is expelled into a cold, bright, noisy environment, and expected to sleep at night-time in a separate bed by themselves. It's a tall order. No wonder many babies struggle with this, crying when they are put down or separated from you in any way.

There are lots of reflexes that newborns have to help them survive and make sense of the world, such as the startle reflex, rooting, sucking and grasping. Throughout the fourth trimester, these reflexes become less automatic and more controlled. The fourth trimester is a great period of discovery for baby, but also for the parents. It can be a real learning curve, getting to know your baby, finding out what they like and what they don't like, feeling happy and elated when you feel like you've kept them happy and settled, lousy and frustrated during the times when your baby has cried lots, despite you trying everything possible to keep them calm. It takes time to distinguish the difference between hunger cries and wind cries, learn your baby's cues, as well as try to look after yourself and indulge in some form of self-care. By the end of the fourth trimester, when your baby is 3–6 months old, you should begin to feel more confident. You will find yourself enjoying watching your baby's personality unravel bit by bit as they learn to smile, coo and become more responsive to their environment.

Small babies don't understand why they have been separated from you and they don't like it. It is a natural instinct for them to want to be held, one of self-preservation – they need to be close to their food source, knowing they are secure and protected. You may also feel an overwhelming urge to hold your baby and be near to them constantly.

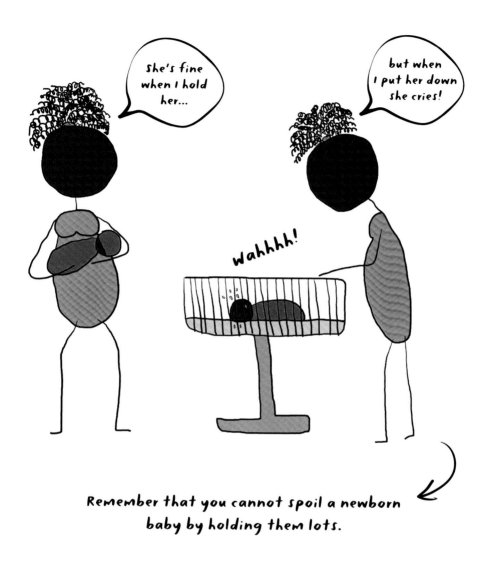

Remember that you cannot spoil a newborn baby by holding them lots.

Those first few months can be super tough – believe me, I've been there a few times. If you are pregnant with your first baby, expect that initially you won't get much done other than caring for your newborn. Try to enlist as much support as you can, and prioritise what really needs to be done at home over what can wait. I found that using a sling to wear my babies was an absolute lifesaver (for more information about slings, see page 243).

The main thing to remember is that the fourth trimester is a journey, one which will have its ups and downs. Remember that with everything you do you are trying your best for your baby, so go easy on yourself.

Registering The Birth

You may have decided on a name for your baby, or you may still be weighing up several names after the birth, while you get to know them.

In the UK you have up to 42 days in which to register the birth in the local district in which your baby was born. As I mentioned on page 177, you should be advised by the midwife who discharges you where to go for registration. Most places require an appointment, so make sure you book in advance.

You will need some form of ID when you register a birth, so take your passport, birth certificate or driving licence (a full list of what's required in the UK is available at *gov.uk/register-birth*). If you are in an opposite-sex relationship, your partner can go on behalf of both of you, as long as you are married or in a civil partnership, otherwise you will need to attend as well. The other parent needs to be there too, to be included on the birth certificate. For same-sex couples, the requirements for registration vary. More details can be found at *gov.uk/register-birth/who-can-register-a-birth*. If you are not in a relationship and want to register as one parent only, you can attend alone to do this.

At the end of the appointment, you will be given a copy of the birth certificate and will have the opportunity to purchase additional copies should you need or want them. Once the birth has been registered, you will be able to officially register your baby at your GP surgery. If, however, you need your newborn to be seen by a GP before you have registered their birth, the surgery will create a temporary ID to allow this.

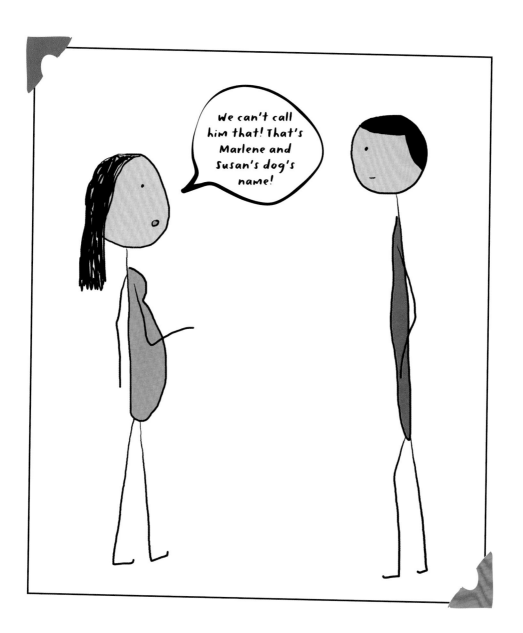

Breastfeeding

Deciding on whether to breastfeed your baby is a personal choice. The term 'breastfeeding' covers any manner in which your baby gets breastmilk, whether that is directly from the breast, via a nasal gastric tube (for preterm and unwell babies), or expressed or donated milk. Knowing what the benefits are, what breastfeeding involves, getting it right and understanding potential problems and how to resolve them, will help you make an informed decision when it comes to feeding your baby.

Understanding the normal function of breasts and milk production

During pregnancy, your breasts go through changes to help them prepare to feed your baby. At some point during the second trimester, your body will start to make a thick substance called colostrum. You may or may not notice a little leaking from your breasts while you are pregnant. Occasionally, colostrum can appear white or even clear, but most of the time it looks yellow. Colostrum, although only produced in tiny amounts, is jam-packed full of nutrients and immunity protection factors. In the first few days, colostrum is all your baby needs, even though it's unlikely you'll be producing much – they'll probably be getting just a few millilitres per feed for the first couple of days, until the volume of milk increases.

Once the baby and placenta are born, several hormonal changes take place.

Progesterone and oestrogen levels drop, and prolactin (the milk-making hormone) increases. As a result of this and regular feeding, the volume of milk increases rapidly in the first few days after birth.

When a baby suckles at the breast, the hormone oxytocin is released from the brain. This in turn causes the ejection of milk through ducts in the breast, out of the nipple. A strange 'fizzing' sensation can sometimes be felt when this happens – this is called the 'let-down' reflex. You will probably find that the let-down reflex is quite strong in the early weeks and months, and may reduce or even disappear as time goes by. You probably won't notice this reflex until you are a few days into your breastfeeding journey. The more frequently a baby feeds from the breast, the more milk will be produced. The relationship between baby, breast and brain is an incredible one, creating a supply and demand situation, so it is important to feed baby often, as your body will only produce what it thinks baby is drinking. Milk supply in normal circumstances is usually established by 3-4 weeks after birth. Between 1 and 6 months, a baby will consume on average 24 ounces (about 700ml) of milk in a twenty-four-hour period. This can vary slightly from baby to baby.

Breastfeeding has several health benefits for both mother and baby:

Baby	Mother
• Reduced risk of infections. • Reduced risk of diarrhoea and vomiting. • Reduced risk of SIDS (sudden infant death syndrome). • Reduced risk of obesity in both infancy and adulthood. • Reduced risk of cardiovascular disease in adulthood.	• Reduced risk of breast cancer. • Reduced risk of ovarian cancer. • Reduced risk of osteoporosis (weak bones). • Reduced risk of cardiovascular disease. • Helps burn calories, thus potentially aids steady postnatal weight loss.

Getting it right

The first thing you need to note is that, to start with, breastfeeding isn't always easy. Some babies will latch onto the breast immediately with no problems and others will take longer to get the hang of it. Some babies will have latch difficulties due to anomalies such as tongue tie (where the piece of skin connecting the baby's tongue to the bottom of their mouth is shorter than usual), and sometimes there are issues due to mother and baby being separated, or as the result of a difficult birth. Ideally, once baby is born, that one hour of golden time for skin-to-skin contact should be given where possible.

This helps to increase levels of oxytocin, keep baby warm and alert them to their awaiting feed.

Getting a good position and latch from the outset is extremely important, as this can prevent nipple pain further down the line. Your midwife should assist and talk you through feeding your baby for the first time after birth. There will also be someone to help you afterwards throughout your time in hospital or in the birth centre. If you have a homebirth, your midwife will ensure baby is feeding before she leaves.

If you're lucky, you may find that having baby skin to skin allows them to crawl up and latch on, known as the 'breast crawl'. Chances are, though, you will need some support if breastfeeding for the first time.

Try these tips for getting a good position and latch:

1. First, set yourself up in a comfortable position. You want to make sure your back is well supported.
2. Bring baby to you, ensuring that their body is in a straight line, with their whole body and head facing the nipple.
3. Support the baby's neck, shoulders and back, allowing them to be able to tilt their head back if necessary.
4. Keeping the baby's nose in line with your nipple, gently brush it over their nose, waiting for them to open their mouth wide. As soon as they do, bring baby swiftly onto the breast, ensuring their lower lip and chin makes contact with the breast first.
5. Your nipple should be pulled up deeply into their mouth.

You should feel baby sucking strongly, but it shouldn't hurt. If it does, de-latch baby by placing a finger into the corner of the mouth to break the suction before removing them. Physical signs that baby is well attached to the breast include:

- The lower lip is curled outwards.
- The chin is touching the breast.
- The mouth is wide open.
- There is more of the areola visible above the baby's top lip than underneath it.

Respond to your baby's feeding cues. When they wake, start rooting around, licking their lips or trying to suck their fist, they are probably ready for a feed. Some babies may find it difficult to switch between pacifier and breast, so avoid a pacifier until breastfeeding is established after the first few weeks.

Remember, babies don't all cry for the breast because they are hungry. Sometimes they want comfort, are tired, unsettled or simply want to be close to you.

Breastfeeding after a caesarean

Many women will worry about breastfeeding after a caesarean. Although it can be trickier to breastfeed after a caesarean due to discomfort from the incision, with the right support and positioning, breastfeeding should be possible.

After a caesarean, skin-to-skin contact can be facilitated to help initiate feeding. The baby can lie across your chest to avoid your wound, but this is something that you will probably need assistance with. Once in the recovery area, you may need help to get into a comfortable position to feed, as your legs will likely still be numb. The first feed is usually recommended within an hour of birth, but that can be delayed a little after a caesarean.

If you are sitting, you may want to put a pillow on your lap to protect your wound. You could always try side-lying with baby, as this means there won't be any

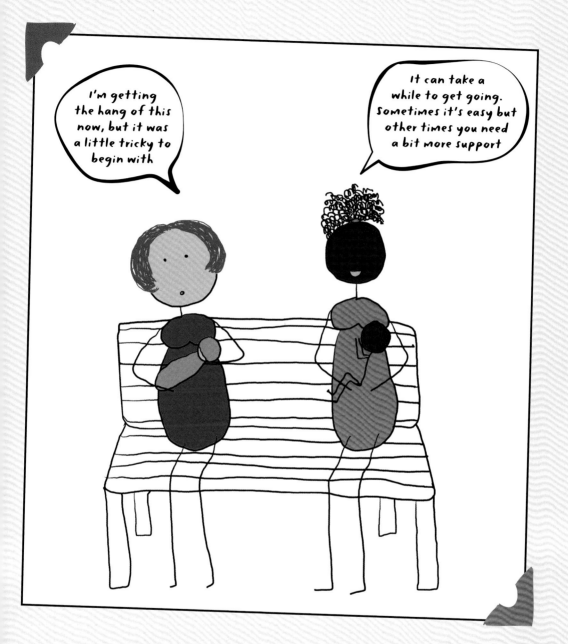

pressure on your abdominal area at all. Make sure you get the help of a midwife, nurse, doula or infant feeding advisor to guide you with positioning and latching. As the days go by, you will begin to feel better and nursing will become easier. When you are home, try to enlist as much help as possible with tasks in the house so that you can just focus on yourself and your baby. Resting, eating, drinking and feeding your baby will be your main focus in the early days!

You may be prescribed some medicines to help with pain and perhaps antibiotics/blood thinners too. You will usually only be prescribed medicines that are safe for breastfeeding, but if in doubt, check with your prescriber.

Pumping or expressing

So, what about expressing breastmilk? You may be wondering how to do it, or if you should. Most babies are able to feed directly from the breast, but there are some circumstances when this may be more challenging. If a baby is premature, is finding latching and sucking difficult, needs time in the neonatal intensive care unit (NICU) for other reasons, or if you are away from your baby (going back to work or having an evening out), expressing is a great way for your baby to get your breastmilk. Some of the ways expressed milk can be given to a baby include: via a syringe, cup, bottle or nasal gastric tube (if they have been given one).

If you need to express milk in the first few days, hand expressing can work better

than a pump for most women. Often, if a breast pump is used too early, the tiny drops of milk that are expressed get caught up in the tubing of the system and don't even reach the bottle. It's better to save using a pump for later on, when the milk volume increases and flows quicker. To hand express, make sure your hands are clean and that you have a sterile container to collect the milk in. Before you begin, gently massage the breast that you are about to express from.

1. Hold one breast, with your fingers and thumb cupped around your breast in a 'C' shape. They should be close to your areola but not touching it.
2. Push your fingers and thumb back into your chest, then compress your breast in between your fingers and thumb, slightly moving them towards your nipple as you do.
3. Release the grip and repeat. After doing this a few times, you should start to notice milk coming out. If you do this in the first day or two after birth, you will probably notice the colostrum coming out slowly in droplets. As the days go by and the milk changes, it should become easier and the milk should flow faster.

If you are in hospital with your baby for a while, you should be able to access a hospital-grade breast pump. A midwife or nurse will show you how to use the pump correctly. If you are exclusively pumping in the early days, you should be expressing regularly throughout the day and night. I would suggest not leaving more than two to three hours between pumping sessions, to ensure you establish and maintain a good supply. There are many manual and electric pumps on the market that you can use at home. If you are hoping to express into a bottle for your baby to be fed by someone else occasionally, it's best to wait until feeding and supply is established before you do this (at around 4 weeks). Once you have expressed your milk, you can store it safely in the fridge in a sterilised container/bottle, or in special breast-milk storage bags for the freezer. The NHS recommends that all items used to express and feed milk should be cleaned with warm soapy water (washing-up liquid is fine). The parts that have come into contact with your milk also need to be sterilised i.e. pump flanges, bottles or cups. You'll find instructions for sterilising on page 197.

Storage guidelines for expressed milk

- **FRIDGE** – Up to 8 days at 4°C or lower. If your fridge temperature is higher than 4°C, use within 3 days.

- **FREEZER** – Up to 6 months at -18°C or lower. If kept in the ice compartment of a fridge, which is less cold, use within 2 weeks. If you have frozen expressed milk, defrost it slowly in the fridge. If you need to give it to baby quickly, however, you can do so by placing the container or bag in a jug of warm water, making sure you shake the bottle before giving it to your baby. Any milk not consumed after one hour should be discarded. Do not refreeze milk that has thawed. Milk stored in the fridge can be warmed up using warm water too.

- If you express and want to feed soon after, you can leave the milk at room temperature for up to six hours, as long as the room temperature isn't higher than 25°C.

Problems with feeding

Breastfeeding is a skill that may take time to learn and isn't always plain-sailing. Sometimes it can take a while to get going and, occasionally, problems can arise after months of fabulous feeding. This section outlines some of the issues faced by some people.

/ SORE OR CRACKED NIPPLES.
Often this is simply as a result of poor attachment to the breast. Get in touch with your care giver: a midwife, infant feeding advisor or lactation consultant will be able to help identify the issue and work out a solution with you. Nipple creams may bring short-term relief.

/ **BREAST ENGORGEMENT.** Primary engorgement is a normal reaction to having a baby. It occurs in the first couple of weeks of birth as the breast tissues swell due to blood and lymph fluids filling the tissues surrounding the alveoli (milk-making glands), in preparation for milk production. The breast is often full, big and hard to the touch. Getting baby to latch on may be difficult, so hand expressing some milk at first, to soften them, may help. Primary engorgement usually lasts for no more than a couple of weeks until your body adjusts to the amount it knows your baby needs. Avoid skipping breastfeeds if you can, as this won't help.

/ **BABY NOT LATCHING PROPERLY.** It's difficult for some babies to latch onto the breast if they don't open their mouths wide enough, if they keep slipping off the breast, or if they don't appear to suckle properly. If you are struggling with getting baby to latch it may be for a number of reasons including tongue tie, birth trauma, cleft palate, medication through labour causing the baby to be sleepy, jaundice, positioning or nipple shape. Sometimes, with flat or inverted nipples it can take a little longer to get feeding going, but with support, patience and perseverance, most babies are able to breastfeed without too much of a problem. It's important to gain practical help with a baby who is not latching properly: a midwife, infant feeding advisor or lactation consultant can examine the baby to identify any physical issues that may be contributing to latching difficulties, and assist you with getting the baby feeding at the breast properly.

/ **MASTITIS AND BLOCKED MILK DUCTS.** Mastitis is a common inflammatory condition that can occur during breastfeeding and lactation, and affects almost one in three women. If this happens, you will probably feel unwell, your breast/breasts may feel warm, heavy and hard, and you may notice a wedge-shaped lump in the breast(s). In light skin, there may be some redness. Mastitis is usually the result of a blocked milk duct that hasn't cleared. Some of the milk banked up behind the blocked duct can be forced into nearby breast tissue, causing the tissue to become inflamed. This inflammation is what we mean by mastitis (infection may or may not be present). If you think you may have mastitis, call your GP or midwife straight away so they can advise you. To keep symptoms from worsening, ensure the sore breast is kept empty by feeding your baby as much as possible, expressing in between feeds if necessary. Drink plenty of fluids and rest as much as you can. Cold packs may help to reduce discomfort, and using a warm compress before feeding may help too. If symptoms are ongoing, antibiotics may be required; most antibiotics can be taken safely while breastfeeding (so no need to 'pump and dump'). It's always worth seeking advice from a lactation consultant or infant feeding advisor to ensure you have baby latched on well, as this will help to prevent mastitis from recurring.

/ **LOW MILK SUPPLY.** Most women will have enough milk to feed their babies. Occasionally some don't, however: this can be down to hormonal issues which affect a very small percentage of the population, not feeding enough from the breast, poor positioning and attachment (subsequently affecting the amount of milk baby is able to take), some medications, excess alcohol consumption or previous breast surgery. (Most people with implants are able to breastfeed, but if you have had breast surgery involving moving the nipple, there may be issues with milk supply.) If you feel your supply is dwindling, the best thing you can do is to feed more often and ensure you are consuming around 3 litres of water per day. If you find drinking lots of fluid difficult, try keeping a water bottle with you throughout the day that you can sip often. You can also try power pumping: power pumping tricks your body into thinking your baby is going through a growth spurt by mimicking cluster feeding (see below), and should therefore act as a trigger to produce more milk. To power pump you need to find a suitable hour in the day and pump on and off over the course of the hour in ten-minute bursts as follows:

- Pump for ten minutes.
- Rest for ten minutes.
- Keep going until the hour is up.

Cluster feeding

Cluster feeding is when the baby feeds extremely frequently due to a growth spurt. They feed often to send a signal to your brain through the breasts to make more milk. During cluster feeding, babies will cry and root around a lot, looking for the breast. Cluster feeding isn't actually

a problem as such, but I've put it in this section as it is one of the reasons many women give up breastfeeding. You're more likely to stick with it if you understand what it is, that it's normal and that it's only temporary. When babies cluster feed, it's easy to mistakenly think the baby is feeding lots and being fussy because you don't have enough milk.

These growth spurts in babies happen at around 7-10 days of age, 2-3 weeks, 3-4 weeks, 3 months, 4 months, 6 months and 9 months of age. During these cluster-feeding growth spurts, be sure to keep hydrated and have snacks handy, as you might be more hungry than usual.

Cluster feeding typically lasts for only a few days before the baby relaxes and gives your body a bit of a break between feeding. Babies don't just cluster feed when going through growth spurts, they can also do it when they are feeling unwell, or unsettled in a new environment. Cluster feeding can really take its toll when you are a new and exhausted mother. It's therefore important to refuel yourself by making sure you're eating well and taking moments to rest whenever possible.

Is baby getting enough milk?

If you are feeding directly from the breast, you won't know the quantities your baby is drinking. So, how do you know if your baby is getting enough milk? There are several things to consider – how the baby feeds, weight, frequency and colour of wet and dirty nappies, and general wellbeing.

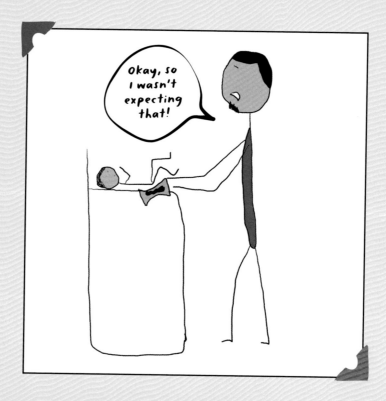

During a breastfeed, you should be able to see and hear your baby swallowing with a rhythmic suck. They tend to take a few rapid sucks initially, to encourage the milk to 'let down' (the reflex that allows breastmilk to flow after tiny nerves are stimulated, sending milk through the breast – it can feel a bit like pins and needles or a fizzing sensation), then sucking slows down to longer, rhythmic sucks. You may find that baby pauses occasionally too. Baby's mouth should be moist and there should be regular wet nappies.

Your baby should appear calm and relaxed during feeds and they will come off on their own at the end. When awake and not feeding, they should appear healthy and alert. If the soft spot at the top of the head (fontanelle) is sunken and their

mouth appears dry, it could be a sign of dehydration.

During the first 2 weeks, your baby will undergo a lot of weight changes, particularly if they're being breastfed. Surprisingly, in the first few days post birth, many babies will lose weight, often because they are getting rid of excess fluids they may have received during labour. If a baby has lost over 10 per cent of their birth weight, support should be given regarding feeding, and an assessment of the baby made. Your midwife will ensure the baby is weighed around days five and ten (see page 200 for more). By 10 days of age, most babies are back to their birth weight, however some can take longer than this. It's important to keep in close contact with your care provider so that they can support you should you have any concerns about weight.

How stools change

Keeping an eye on the baby's urine and stool output is key. In the first twenty-four hours, don't expect many dirty nappies. A baby will usually pass urine a couple of times and pass meconium once – their first bowel movement. Meconium is a dark, thick, tar-like substance that has formed in the baby's bowel during pregnancy.

As the baby feeds on milk, the colour and consistency of their poo changes. By day two or three, there should be some visible changes in colour as it appears greener. It should be brown/orange tinged on day four or five, and yellow/runny by day five or six. Expect one or two bowel movements per day at the start, and by the end of the first week, you'll probably find you're changing around six to twelve nappies per day! This may go on for some time, until they start eating solid food at around 6 months old. Many breastfed babies hit a point at around 4–6 weeks of age where they don't poo as often. This can be alarming, but it's usually nothing to worry about. Some babies can go many days without passing a stool. It is thought that this is because all of the breastmilk consumed is being used, so there is very little waste. If you have other concerns about your baby however, or it's been more than 7 days since they opened their bowels, contact your health visitor or GP for advice.

This chart is a guideline on how much your baby will be eating, peeing and pooing in the first few days. This is based on a healthy full-term baby of average weight:

	Wet	Poo	Breast	Formula
First 24 hrs	1+	1+	3–12 feeds	Up to 1oz (30ml) 2–3 hourly*
Day 2	2+	1+	8–12 feeds	Up to 2oz (60ml) 2–3 hourly*
Day 3	3+	1+	8–12 feeds	Up to 2oz (60ml) 2–3 hourly*
Day 4	4+	1+	8–12 feeds	Up to 2oz (60ml) 2–3 hourly*
Day 5	5+	2+	8–12 feeds	Up to 2oz (60ml) 2–3 hourly*

*GUIDELINE ONLY, BABIES' NEEDS VARY

Formula Feeding

If a baby is not being fed breastmilk, the alternative is to feed them formula. Formula milk is an infant food usually made from cow's milk. It comes in a powdered form to mix with water, or pre-made and ready to drink.

If you choose to formula-feed your baby, it's important to know how to make feeds correctly to ensure your baby receives the right amount of milk. Pre-made ready-to-drink formula takes the worry out of making it up correctly, but it is more expensive. It is handy to have, however, if you are on the go. 'First infant formula' is the only formula you need to give your baby unless your doctor has advised you otherwise. There is no evidence that 'hungry baby' milks settle babies more or help them to sleep longer.

If you buy powdered formula milk, be sure to make up the feeds exactly as the instructions state. As a general rule, the steps to making up a formula milk bottle are as follows:

1. Boil kettle and allow water to cool for twenty minutes. Water needs to still be hot enough to kill any potential bacteria in the milk powder.
2. Wash hands and grab a bottle that has been sterilised.
3. Pour in the water first – this is extremely important. Putting the powder in first can distort the water/powder ratio. Fill to the level you have decided to give. Most bottles will display fluid ounces. Check the packet to see how many scoops of powder to add.
4. Add the powder to the bottle, ensuring you flatten and level the scoop off first. There is usually a plastic spatula in the container to carry this out.
5. Screw on the sterilised lid and teat, shake well and test the temperature on the inside of your wrist before giving it to your baby. Any unused milk should be discarded within two hours.

Ideally, each feed should be made up as and when it is required, to reduce the chance of bacteria multiplying in the milk.

It should feel lukewarm and not hot. If you have no choice but to store a feed, place the covered bottle in the back of a fridge for no more than twenty-four hours. Once out of the fridge, it can be gently warmed up in a pan of warm water and should be drunk within two hours (discard any leftover milk).

Sterilising bottles

Babies' immune systems are not as developed as an older child's or adult's, so sterilising bottles is essential to prevent bacteria multiplying and causing your baby to become unwell. There are several ways you can sterilise your baby's feeding equipment, such as using a cold-water sterilising system, steam sterilising, and sterilising by boiling. Putting bottles in a dishwater may clean the bottles but it won't sterilise them as the water is not hot enough. Cold-water sterilisers use tablets that dissolve in the water, which subsequently kills any bacteria it comes into contact with. Sterilising with steam or boiling water relies on high heat levels to kill the bacteria.

Before you begin to sterilise, wash your hands thoroughly and ensure all the surfaces you use are clean. Clean all parts of the bottle and teat in hot soapy water (just as you would with cutlery or dishes), with the help of a bottle brush, removing all visible traces of milk. Rinse each part in clean, cool water before sterilising. For cold water and steam sterilising, follow the manufacturer's instructions on the tablet box and steam-steriliser insert. If you decide to sterilise by boiling, follow these simple steps:

- Put all the cleaned bottle parts in a pan of boiling water for at least ten minutes.
- Ensure that all items are covered with the water.
- Never leave hot pans unattended, particularly if you have children present.

Remove the bottles from the water with kitchen tongs rather than your hands if the water is hot! Leave the sterilised bottles somewhere clean until ready to use. If you are not using them immediately, assemble them fully, with the teat covered by the lid. Don't rinse with tap water before use, as that will make them unsterile again.

Hold your baby close to you when bottle feeding to promote bonding and warmth. Avoid leaving your baby with the bottle propped up for feeding, as this can be a choking hazard.

Combination feeding

If you are not able to, or don't wish to exclusively breastfeed, you may decide that feeding your baby both breastmilk and formula works best for you. This can be direct from the breast, combined with formula bottle feeds, or expressed milk in a bottle along with formula feeds. If combi feeding feels right, find a routine that you and baby are happy with, remembering that your breastmilk supply will decrease the longer the breasts go without being emptied of milk. Some parents I've cared for have opted to combi feed: perhaps mostly breastfeeding and using one bottle of formula in the day, or giving baby a 50/50 amount of breastmilk and formula.

Visitors

When a baby is born, family and friends can become incredibly excited and eager to meet the new arrival.

I would always suggest limiting visitors, initially. Of course, most of us will have parents and close siblings visit us at some point but too many people can be overwhelming, especially when we are trying to establish feeding, may be bleeding, uncomfortable with stitches and exhausted. When you decide to allow visitors is totally up to you. It's always good to set boundaries though, as it can become stressful, especially when you are trying to rest, recover, bond with your baby and learn how to feed them. You may also find it overwhelming if there are too many people handling your baby.

Be clear from the beginning about who can visit and when. You may decide that, in the first few days, you only want the baby's grandparents with you. Find a safe space in your home that you can retreat to if need be: you may feel like you need to lie down, have a rest, or feed the baby without the distraction of conversation or noise.

Most visitors will be happy to help out in any way they can. Don't feel afraid to ask someone to bring over some milk, to put the kettle on, make you a snack or hold the baby while you shower. Undoubtedly, there will be times when a visitor is holding your baby and the baby starts to cry. For most new mums, the initial thought is 'my baby needs me'. Some visitors are in tune with this and will hand them straight back, while others will try to settle the baby themselves, perhaps just wanting to be helpful and give you a break. If you are in this situation, a simple, 'Oh, pass her here, let me go feed her,' will usually suffice.

Babies have a wonderful scent that most people love. Visitors will cuddle and rock your baby, but it's important that they don't kiss them on their face or lips (some people carry the herpes simplex virus which causes cold sores, even if they have never had a cold sore. Although harmless in adults, it can cause severe problems in babies). Offer visitors some antibacterial gel for their hands too, when they arrive.

Your partner can also help with guarding your space as a family during this time, answering phone calls from keen friends and family, letting them know what visiting arrangements you have made. Sometimes being firm on timings helps prevent people

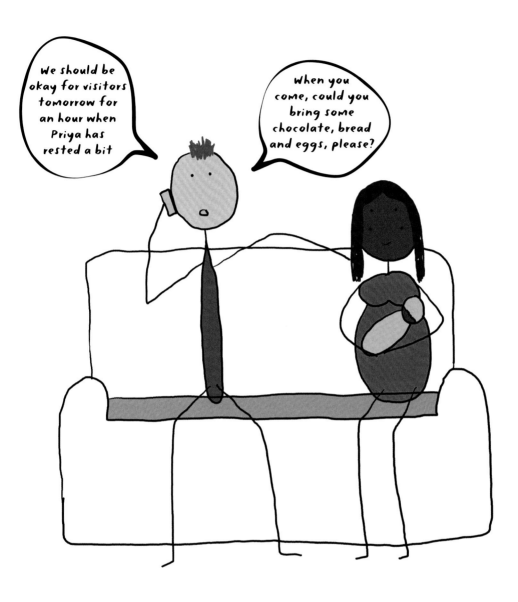

from overstaying their welcome. When you've just had a baby, having a hoard of visitors arrive at 10 a.m. and stay until 6 p.m. is often just too much. Offering visiting timeframes is a good way to deter this: saying, for example, 'Sure, pop in briefly between 2-3 p.m.' can let a visitor know not to stay too long.

Ultimately, everyone is different. Whether you want no visitors or are happy with several is a personal choice. Whatever you decide, make sure that you put your recovery and your baby's new journey at the forefront.

Postnatal Care From Professionals

After you have had your baby, there will be follow-up care from health professionals who work within the local community. They will check your physical and mental wellbeing, as well as provide support during your transition into motherhood.

In the UK, you can usually expect a home visit by a midwife the day after you arrive home (do check with your midwife though, as regional postnatal community services vary). During this appointment, the midwife will ask about your first night, check how you are physically by feeling your abdomen, ask about blood loss, ask how your appetite has been, check perineal healing and more. They will also check on baby by examining them fully and asking you about their feeding and bowel movements. In addition, the midwife will give you information about when and where the rest of your postnatal appointments will be.

As standard, you can expect to see a midwife again around day five and day ten. On day five the baby is weighed and offered a newborn blood spot test which is part of a national screening programme for babies. It checks for a number of rare disorders, many of which have a better prognosis if caught early. More information about the blood spot test can be found at *nhs.uk/conditions/baby/newborn-screening/blood-spot-test.*

Your baby will also be weighed on day five and again on day ten. If all appears to be going well with both you and baby, you will be discharged from midwifery care and transferred to the care of a 'health visitor'. Health visitors are there to support families with children up to the age of 5 years. They usually provide a couple of visits in the first couple of months and will talk to you about the immunisation programme, your mental health, local support groups and answer any other concerns you may have.

At around 6 weeks after the birth, you will be advised to book an appointment with your GP to check on your wellbeing, talk about contraception, and also to perform a general examination of the baby. During the first 10 days, if you have any concerns regarding you or your baby, contact the maternity unit for advice. After this time, when you can be discharged from the care of the community team, your GP will be the one to contact.

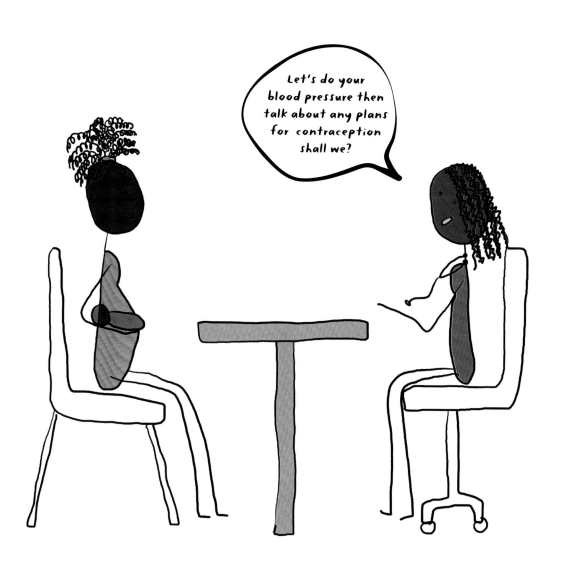

Recovery And Self-care

The first few days and weeks after having a baby can be wonderful, exhausting and anxiety-inducing all at the same time!

After a vaginal birth

Your road to recovery after a vaginal birth will depend on your physical healing, good support at home and self-care. Focus on your recovery and caring for baby. Your partner can help you by ensuring you rest where possible and taking care of household tasks. Setting up a comfy spot on the sofa can be useful, as some days you may feel stuck there snuggling with your baby, particularly if you are breastfeeding. Have plenty of cushions, drinks, snacks, the remote control and your phone charger within reaching distance.

For physical recovery, it may help to have a peri spray bottle to squirt warm water on the perineum. Even if you don't have a perineal tear, it still may be a little tender. If you did have a tear or an episiotomy during birth, you may worry about the healing process but most perineums heal just fine after some time and care. Small first-degree tears are usually left to heal without stitches. Allow at least 2 weeks for your perineum to start feeling better. If you have a deeper tear, or an episiotomy that required stitches, it may take a few more days to heal. Most sutures are dissolvable, so you don't have to worry about having them removed – you may find they just start coming away naturally after a week or so.

Try not to worry about going to the toilet for a number two, either – your stitches won't burst open! To make it easier to go, drink plenty of water and eat lots of vegetables to avoid constipation. You may even be prescribed a laxative, depending on the grade of your tear. Shower or bathe at least once a day and avoid soap or bubbles. When you have finished, pat the area dry rather than rubbing it. Simple paracetamol or ibuprofen can be helpful. Begin pelvic floor exercises ('Kegels' – see page 212) as soon as you feel able to – this will help to strengthen the pelvic floor and prevent continence problems later in life. Ultimately, time is a healer and within a couple of weeks you will find that your perineum feels much better. If at any stage when you go home you develop a high temperature or find that the pain gets worse, seek advice from your midwife. You can expect bleeding to continue after birth for 2–8 weeks on average. It will be quite heavy to begin with, settling down within a week or so to a lighter flow. If you are bleeding heavily, soaking through more than one pad an hour, contact your maternity unit to speak to a midwife for advice. Your abdomen will more than likely still look pretty swollen. It takes some time for the uterus to shrink back down to its pre-pregnancy state. Go easy on yourself; your body has been through some incredible changes.

After a caesarean

Looking after yourself and recovering from a caesarean is somewhat different to self-care after a vaginal birth, and recovery usually takes longer. Everyone's postnatal experience after a caesarean will be unique, but keep in mind that a caesarean is major abdominal surgery, so your body will need sufficient time to heal. If you know you are going to have a caesarean, it's easier to be prepared and get things in place for postnatal recovery (such as batch-cooking), but if you have an unplanned one, it can take you by surprise a little!

Most people are in hospital for 1–4 days after a caesarean and, depending on hospital guidelines or risk factors, you may be offered compression socks and blood-thinning injections to administer yourself at home for a few days. This helps prevent blood clots while you are not particularly mobile. Take one step at a time – some may tell you how they were running around within hours of surgery with little discomfort, but not everyone has the same experience. Many will find walking around a lot after surgery very uncomfortable – I did! Try to gently mobilise when you can though, as it helps prevent blood clots.

If you arrive home with the dressing still in place and have been told to remove it yourself, an easy way to do this is in the shower. Getting the dressing wet makes the sticky gauze easy to peel away, without pulling at your hair. Your community midwife will visit you at home after the birth and remove the stitches, unless they are dissolvable; ask what kind you have before leaving the hospital. Your care provider will give you information on when to do this. Keep an eye out for any oozing coming through the dressing and, once it's removed, contact your care provider if you notice signs of infection, including a high temperature of over 37.5°C, increased pain around the scar, or an oozing or gaping wound. As the wound heals, you may develop a small bump where the skin meets and this is usually scar tissue. When it's totally healed (which takes about 6 weeks), massage it gently to encourage it to flatten. During the healing period, you may notice itchiness and numbness which may take some time to disappear, or you might notice that there is always a slight section of numbness along the scar.

Enlist plenty of support, assigning physically-demanding jobs to your partner (or another helping hand). Avoid lifting anything heavier than your baby for the first few weeks. If you have a toddler, encourage them to sit with you for cuddles rather than lifting them.

Driving after a caesarean is not advised for 6 weeks. Driving before this time may break the terms of your insurance, so check your policy before heading off on your first postnatal outing as the designated driver.

Emotions After The Birth

The birth of a baby is the most amazing time in a woman's life, right? For most, yes, but for many women, it just doesn't feel that way.

Around 80 per cent of women will experience intense emotional change after the birth. This happens regardless of the birth experience or other external factors, but we know that stress, traumatic birth, issues with breastfeeding and relationship problems can increase the risk of postnatal depression. For many, their baby is born and the rush of love is instant; for others, this can take time and it's easy to feel extremely guilty for feeling this way.

Often, emotional change manifests itself in the form of the 'day-three blues'. The 'day-three blues' doesn't actually mean you'll feel down on day three after birth, it just happens to occur quite commonly around that time. Bursting into tears easily, experiencing mood swings and feeling overwhelmed are perfectly normal. You are exhausted from lack of sleep and are trying to recover from the birth experience: coupled with rapid hormone changes and the responsibility of looking after a newborn, it's not surprising that many women experience the tense emotions of the 'day-three blues'. This feeling usually improves within a few days, or after a couple of weeks at most.

Sometimes, the feelings commonly associated with 'day-three blues' can escalate, become prolonged and interfere with daily life. If you are feeling persistently down, overwhelmed, tearful, depressed, guilty, fearful, detached from the baby, disinterested in daily events or just not quite yourself, and it's ongoing, then talk to someone about it – this person can be someone close to you or a health professional. Postnatal depression (PND) is a common mental-health illness which women can recover from best if it's recognised and treated promptly. Partners are not exempt from PND. Tommy's charity estimates that as many as 1 in 10 men suffer from some form of depression during their partner's pregnancy or after the birth. Mental health charities such as MIND have resources for partners experiencing depression in and around pregnancy.

Similar to antenatal depression, PND can occur in anyone, but it is more likely to present in people who have a previous history of depression, parents who have little support, bereaved parents, people who've had a traumatic birth experience or have experienced/are experiencing domestic abuse. PND can occur at any time within the

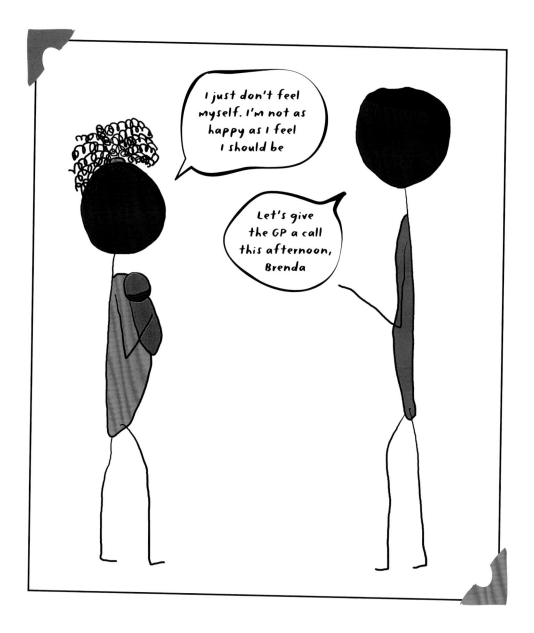

first year after birth, with many not realising they have it, due to symptoms creeping up over time. Keep an eye on how you're feeling, be kind to yourself and seek help if you need to from friends, family, your health visitor or a local support group.

Postnatal Complications

After giving birth, it's really easy to be so focused on caring for your baby that you can become distracted from looking after your own health. Health problems can occasionally occur in the weeks following birth, so it's good to know what to look out for. Help is always just a phone call away, should you or anyone close to you notice anything out of the ordinary.

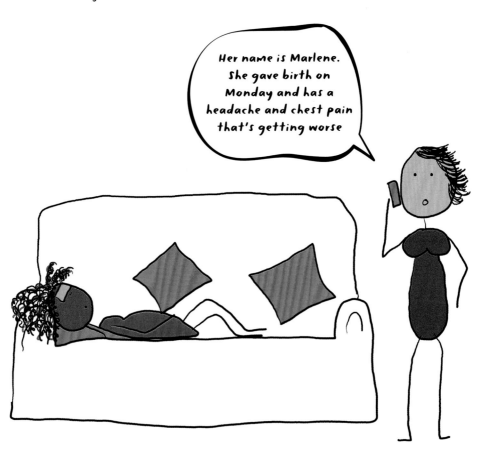

After birth, it's common to experience tiredness and discomfort, and you're likely to feel achy and bruised: as I have already mentioned, you may experience afterpains or perineal soreness. So, how can you tell if there is a problem?

The most serious complications to be aware of are:

- Infection or sepsis – from a caesarean or perineal wound, or mastitis.
- Blood pressure problems – such as HELPP syndrome, a more severe form of pre-eclampsia.
- Complications from pre-existing conditions such as heart disease.
- Postpartum haemorrhage.
- Blood clots – sometimes these can occur in the legs, particularly after long periods of immobility.
- Puerperal or post-partum psychosis – a severe mental-health disorder affecting people who have recently given birth. It usually starts suddenly, within days or weeks of birth. The symptoms can be scary for some, varying widely, and can change rapidly: they can include depression, confusion, hallucinations and delusions. Delusional behaviour is usually noticed initially by the partner.

Sometimes, risk factors for postnatal complications can be identified during pregnancy, which means either treatment can be put in place prior to the baby's birth, or at least you know exactly what to look out for. An example would be giving someone with a high-risk score for developing blood clots blood-thinning injections post birth. If pre-eclampsia was diagnosed in pregnancy, blood pressure may be monitored postnatally too. Other times, however, postnatal complications can just occur out of the blue. Don't worry – many postnatal complications can be treated successfully if they are identified early. Pay attention to your wellbeing and always reach out for advice if you don't feel right.

Seek emergency 999 help if you have:

- Severe chest pain or sudden shortness of breath, or difficulty breathing.
- Severe sudden head pain.
- Seizures.
- Thoughts of harming yourself or your baby.

Seek advice from your care provider if you have:

- An area of your leg that is painful, swollen and warm to the touch. In light skin complexions there may also be redness.
- Bleeding and soaking through more than one pad an hour, or large blood clots the size of a satsuma or bigger.
- A wound that isn't healing.
- A temperature of 38°C or higher.
- A headache that gets worse or doesn't improve, even after taking an analgesic.

Always trust your instinct and remember there will always be someone to offer you help and advice after the birth of your baby, on a twenty-four-hour basis.

Sex And Contraception

When you decide to have sex post birth is totally up to you and when you feel comfortable. Some health professionals are old-school and advise waiting 6 weeks, but ultimately it really is at your discretion!

You might want to consider which contraception you prefer to use before you resume having sex. I would suggest using a condom if you do have sex before you have arranged any longer-term contraception such as the pill or coil.

Around 6 weeks after birth, you can discuss longer-term birth-control options with your doctor or GP if using condoms indefinitely is not suitable for you.

Having sexual intercourse for the first time after giving birth can be nerve-racking, so only do it when you are ready. If you are tense and anxious, it can make sex difficult. Consider using lubrication if necessary, as postpartum hormones can cause vaginal dryness, especially with breastfeeding. If you have had a caesarean, you may not have any vaginal or perineal trauma but you will still have a healing abdominal wound. Perhaps try having intercourse in a position other than missionary, that won't put excess pressure on it.

If you have any perineal wounds that are taking a while to heal, or you are getting over an infection in the uterus, vagina or perineum, it would be best to wait until you are totally healed.

Have you heard about breastfeeding being a form of contraceptive? While it is true that exclusive breastfeeding may delay the release of an egg, thus preventing pregnancy in some women, it's not totally guaranteed. Breastfeeding mothers may find their periods take longer to resume – anywhere from 6 weeks to over a year for some. I would still not rely on it 100 per cent as a form of contraception, unless you are happy to have your babies back to back, which is what some families want to do! It is worthwhile noting, though, that falling pregnant too soon after giving birth does put you at an increased risk of preterm birth, not to mention exhaustion. I recommend waiting for at least 9 months to give your body time to recover before trying to conceive again.

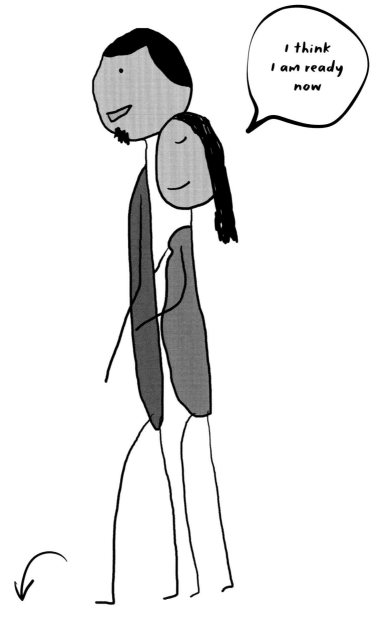

Only have sex when you are ready and feel
100 per cent relaxed.

Diet

Eating well postnatally is essential to ensure your body is fuelled for daily activities, including caring for a newborn and breastfeeding.

Thankfully, once your baby is born, there aren't as many restrictions on what you can eat. If you fancy that rare steak, go for it (although personally, I prefer mine well done!).

For many, there is a huge desire to lose weight quickly after having a baby. Be gentle on yourself! Focus on consuming the right foods to nourish your body to support postnatal recovery, milk production and general wellbeing.

Any form of crash dieting, whether it's restricting either calories or carbohydrates, is not a good idea. A steady supply of carbohydrates is actually necessary for new mothers: they support hormone regulation and mental health, boost energy, breastmilk production and more. If you are concerned about weight you've gained while pregnant, give yourself time. It took you 9 months to grow your baby, so allow your body at least 9 months to recover. If you eat a well-balanced diet, without being too restrictive, you will shed much of the excess anyway. The key is patience, good meals and a bit of self-kindness.

When you are breastfeeding, you are likely to need between 200 and 500 more calories per day than you consumed pre-pregnancy. Your body will tell you when you are hungry, but it's always ideal to have a healthy snack (i.e. fruit, yoghurt, nuts, oat bars) and water handy when you are feeding. Your thirst will increase and so should your fluid intake – to about 3 litres a day. This will help to keep you hydrated and maintain a good milk supply. Hydration can vary from person to person, so thirst should be your real guide. Drink according to thirst and keep an eye on the colour of your urine – if it's clear or very pale yellow, it's likely that you are hydrated. If your urine is dark yellow, it could mean that dehydration is setting in and you need to reach for some water.

Appropriate caloric intake varies from woman to woman depending on body size, activity levels and other variations. Ideally, you want to have a nutritious, varied diet rather than focusing too much on counting calories. Prioritise nourishing your body with healthy sources of protein, fruit, vegetables, fibre-rich carbs, and good-fat foods such as nuts, seeds and avocados.

It is recommended to take a 10mcg vitamin D supplement if you're breastfeeding

Vitamin D is important, as it helps your bones absorb calcium and therefore plays a major role in the bone health of both adults and children. Vitamin D primarily comes from sunlight but is also found in foods such as oily fish (fish like salmon, sardines and mackerel), red meat and some breakfast cereals. It is hard, however, to get enough vitamin D from food alone, hence the recommendation for supplements. If your baby is exclusively breastfeeding, i.e. without any formula top-ups, it's recommended that you give your baby a vitamin D supplement too, of 8.5–10mcg. These can be found in the form of drops in most chemists and some health-food shops.

Are there any foods that should be avoided postnatally?

While advice around what you should and shouldn't eat after birth is in general more relaxed than eating during pregnancy, there are still some dietary points to consider:

/ **CAFFEINE**, when consumed in large quantities, can make your baby restless, affecting their sleep. This is because small amounts can filter through to your breastmilk. It is advised to limit your caffeine intake to around 200ml of caffeinated drinks a day: equivalent to one to two cups of coffee per day. Avoid energy drinks which are high in caffeine (and sugar) and perhaps consider opting for caffeine-free alternatives when choosing a drink.

/ **DRINKING ALCOHOL** in small amounts is unlikely to have a significant impact on your baby, as when drunk in moderation only small quantities will enter your milk. Some people, however, prefer to steer clear of alcohol altogether when breastfeeding. Limit yourself to the occasional drink every now and then. Drinking to intoxication is likely to have a detrimental impact on your ability to properly care for your baby, regardless of whether you are breastfeeding or not.

Exercise:
pelvic floor and abdominal exercises

You may be wondering when you can start exercising after having a baby. The answer varies from person to person, and what type of birth you have had. If you have had a caesarean, you will probably need to wait a little longer to start physical exercise than if you have had a vaginal birth.

Pelvic floor exercises should be started as soon as possible after birth for women who have had either a vaginal or caesarean birth. By carrying out pelvic floor exercises every day, which help to strengthen the muscles around your bladder, vagina and rectum, you are less likely to suffer from incontinence, prolapse and problems with sexual intercourse.

You don't need any special tools or space to do pelvic floor exercises – they can be practised in any position, lying down, standing or sitting, and you can do them anywhere and at any time! A good time to do your pelvic floor exercises is when you're on the toilet, because this means that you are doing them several times a day.

Here are the steps to performing a pelvic floor exercise, also known as 'Kegels':

- Imagine you are holding in wind from your back passage and squeeze.
- At the same time, imagine you are also stopping the flow of urine by squeezing around your vagina and bladder.
- Hold for as long as you can, but no longer than ten seconds.
- Aim to repeat this ten times, three times per day.
- Aim to build up to ten repeats of each exercise, at least three times a day.

Try doing one now while you're reading this book – you'll be surprised at how easy it is!

Low-impact exercise post birth, such as walking, pilates and yoga, is generally safe to start as soon as you feel able to after a vaginal birth. This may be after a few weeks. If you have had a caesarean, wait until your 6-week postnatal appointment with your GP before you return to exercise at the same level as you were doing pre-pregnancy. When

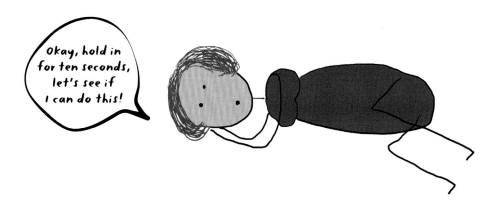

you do start to exercise, build up slowly, starting with the low-impact exercises first. In some cases, your GP may recommend you wait for at least 12 weeks before starting any high-impact exercises, for example running, team sports or weight training.

Resuming physical exercise after you have given birth is a good way to strengthen your abdominal muscles, back and core. It's common for the abdominal muscles to separate during pregnancy due to the pressure of the growing uterus – this separation is known as diastasis recti, or divarication. The gap is often identified by being able to place two fingers in between the muscles. They usually return to normal by the time your baby is 8 weeks old, but occasionally it can take longer. If you notice that there is still an obvious gap after this time, visit your GP, who may be able to refer you to a physiotherapist.

Some stronger abdominal exercises such as crunches can help with strength and fitness, but don't try them until 6 weeks after birth, unless advised otherwise by your care provider.

A simple abdominal strengthening exercise

1. Lie down on one side, with your knees drawn up slightly.
2. Relax your abdomen and breathe in slowly. As you exhale, use your muscles to draw in your lower abdomen as if you were narrowing your waistline.
3. Hold for ten seconds, then release.
4. Repeat this up to ten times, as long as you feel comfortable.

Postnatal Hair Changes

Do you know that your hair can change texture after birth? Some people have reported that their hair has become curlier or straighter after children. In my case, as I've got older, each time I have a child, my curl pattern changes drastically!

Many people notice hair loss after pregnancy, but did you know why? Normally, around 85–95 per cent of your hair is in the growth phase at any point in time, but the hormonal changes during pregnancy stimulate an increase in the percentage of hairs in the growth phase. As a result, many women enjoy thicker hair during pregnancy, as more hairs than normal are growing and fewer than normal are resting or shedding.

With the birth of your baby (and the hormonal changes that accompany birth), a larger number of hairs than normal enter the resting phase. Since the resting phase is followed by hair shedding (and regrowth), new mothers will experience greater than normal hair loss once the resting phase ends.

Postnatal hair loss commonly starts at around 3 months after birth. The amount of time between childbirth and the onset of shedding corresponds to the length of the resting phase of hair growth (between 1 and 6 months, with an average of 3 months).

The hair loss can seem more extreme if you have long hair. Most women will return to their usual hair growth cycle within 6 months, or between 6 and 12 months after birth.

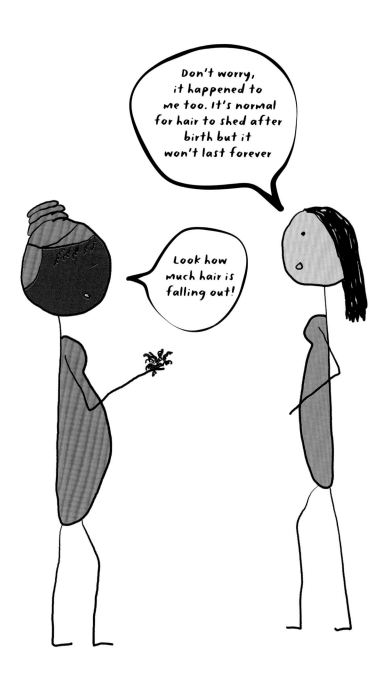

Out And About:
going out for the first
time with baby

Different cultures and traditions have different ideas on when to go out with your baby and there is an abundance of conflicting advice about when is the best time to take your baby out of the house. Ultimately, when you decide to take your baby out is totally up to you.

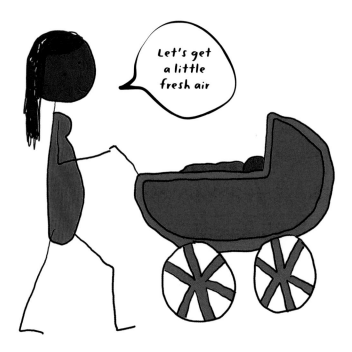

If you are having your first baby and there is no real rush to take baby out, you may want to enjoy as much recovery time as possible at home in those early days. If you have a child that is school age, you may find yourself having to do school runs when your baby is only a few days old, especially if you have little support or your partner is self-employed and has to return to work soon after the birth. The key thing is to only go out if you feel well. If you are in a lot of discomfort, don't go out. If you have stitches, it will probably take several days before mobilising becomes more comfortable.

You don't have to stay indoors with your baby until they have had their first vaccinations, contrary to popular belief – just ensure that your baby is dressed appropriately for the weather.

My key tips for you when you decide to venture out:

- **Take your time** – Leaving the house with a baby is very different to leaving by yourself. Putting pressure on yourself to get out at a certain time is likely to stress you out, especially when your baby decides they want to be fed or need a nappy change as you are about to leave!
- **Get yourself ready first** – Have a shower and dress as they are napping, or when someone is with them. Make sure you have something to eat and drink before organising what you will need for your journey.
- **Start small** – When you first go out, make it a small journey. This could be just a stroll around the block with baby in a pram or carrier.
- **Don't take too much with you** – A couple of nappies, a change of clothes, a muslin square or bib, a sanitary pad and a bag should suffice. Don't forget a bottle for your baby if you're not breastfeeding, and a drink and snack for you.
- **Go to a comfortable place** – After your initial short venture out, you may decide you want to go to another public setting such as a coffee shop or restaurant. Choose somewhere close by that has baby-friendly facilities and a comfortable space to be able to breastfeed.

Dressing a baby appropriately

It's important to dress your baby according to the weather, to prevent them from overheating or becoming too cold. A good way to gain a sense of your baby's temperature is to feel their chest or back. It should always be warm to the touch (for more on checking baby's temperature, see page 221).

Layering your baby's clothing is the best way to dress them. This traps heat in between each layer, making it easier to cool them down or warm them up by adding or removing layers where necessary. Thin cotton clothes are best for a baby's skin, starting with a short-sleeved bodysuit underneath a sleeper onesie. Add as required for cold weather. This may involve popping a snowsuit and hat on baby in extreme weather, and finishing off by covering baby with blankets outside. Be cautious of overheating with too many layers on in warm venues. As soon as you enter a warm building or return home after being out in the cold, remove the snowsuit or any winter layers.

When the temperature is 24°C and above, a single layer is often enough. This may be a long-sleeved onesie or, in extreme heat, a short-sleeved one. It's important to protect your baby from the sun by keeping them in the shade. Most sunscreens cannot be used on a baby's skin until they are over 6 months old. Protect baby by ensuring they are never in direct sunlight. You can purchase prams with wide hoods or parasols. In this sort of heat, never cover your baby's pram with a blanket/towel etc. as this can trap heat and cause your baby's temperature to rise rapidly.

Car seats

If you travel in a car with a baby, you must use a car seat for safety. Most manufacturers make their seats according to the i-size regulations – these can be found at *childcarseats.org.uk/choosing-using.*

Some pram systems allow a car seat to be connected as the carriage, making it easier to remove them from the car to the pram. Newborn babies shouldn't spend more than two hours at a time in a car seat and, where possible, you should sit with them in the rear of the car to ensure they are comfortable, providing you're not driving.

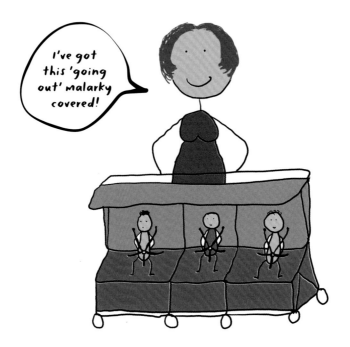

"

Newborn babies cry on average for about two and a half hours each day, on and off. This may seem like a lot but it's their only form of communication.

"

How To Tell If Baby Is Unwell

In situations where a baby may become unwell, it's important to seek the appropriate help. Even if some of the physical observations listed here look okay but you are still concerned, always trust your instinct and call your doctor for advice. You know your baby better than anyone. The information in this section will help you to have a basic understanding of what observations are normal in newborns and babies under 1 year.

Muscle tone and colour

Babies should have a healthy colour, depending on their normal complexion. Any blue tinge to their body, lips or face, known as cyanosis, is not normal and needs to be checked out right away. In darker-skinned babies this may be more difficult to identify, so always check the inside of their mouth and tongue for signs of cyanosis. Some newborn infants can have very pale hands and feet, which is normal in the early days. Healthy babies should have good muscle tone. They usually have their knees bent and fists clenched, unless sleeping. A baby that has suddenly become floppy or lacks good muscle tone should be assessed without delay.

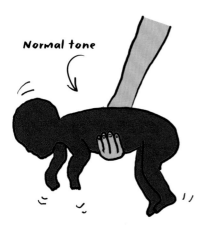

Normal tone

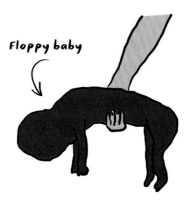

Floppy baby

Temperature

A normal temperature for a baby should be between 36.4 and 37.5°C. You can take your baby's temperature using a digital thermometer under the armpit. If your baby has a temperature of 38°C or more, and has a rash or is under 3 months old, seek advice from your doctor or call 111 if it is out of hours. If your baby is over 3 months old and has a temperature of 38–39°C, you may want to consider giving them a paracetamol syrup to try to bring their temperature down. Plenty of water (or milk if not yet 6 months old) will also help. Most fevers are caused by a virus which is self-resolving. If a fever hasn't resolved within forty-eight hours, seek advice from a doctor. If any child of any age has a temperature of over 39°C, seek advice from a doctor ASAP.

Breathing and heart rate

Breathing too fast or too slow can be a cause for concern in infants, especially in the presence of other unusual symptoms. If you're concerned, you can assess this yourself initially. Count each breath in and out as one breath over the course of one minute to get your baby's respiratory rate. You can do the same for your baby's heart rate by placing your hand on their chest and counting each beat. Baby's heart rates are faster than adults, even when they are born. The normal values for breathing and heart rates are as follows:

Age	Average heart rate (bpm)	Average respiratory rate (rpm)
0–1 year	110–160	40
1–2 years	100–150	35
3–4 years	95–140	30
5–11 years	80–120	25

Signs of meningitis

Meningitis is an inflammation of the membranes around the brain and spinal cord. Babies in the UK are now routinely offered the MenB vaccine in infancy, but it's worthwhile knowing the signs to look out for if they haven't yet had the vaccine:

- Fever and cold hands and feet.
- Refusing food and vomiting.
- Fretful, dislike being handled.
- Drowsy, floppy, unresponsive.
- Rapid breathing or grunting.

- Pale, blotchy skin. Spots/rash that doesn't fade when pressed with a glass.
- Unusual cry, moaning.
- Tense, bulging fontanelle (soft spot on the head).

If you think your baby may have meningitis, call 999.

Baby Skin

As your baby adjusts to their new environment, you may notice several changes in their skin.

Some babies are born coated in a white waxy substance called vernix. It's an amazingly rich protective layer that prevents the skin from damage while in the womb. Could you imagine spending 9 months in a bath? Your skin would be pretty wrinkly, wouldn't it? Vernix is usually most visible in babies that are born at or just before their estimated due date. Newborn skin undergoes a number of adaptions to the outside world in terms of pH and hydration and vernix helps to regulate these changes, so it's worthwhile not bathing baby too soon. If your baby is born with a layer of vernix, use it as a moisturiser, gently rubbing it into their skin as opposed to wiping it off.

Some babies may have dry, flaky skin, particularly those that are born later than expected. This is usually temporary and doesn't normally require you to put anything on it.

There are several types of birthmark that may make an appearance on your baby's skin, too. Blue-grey spots (or slate-grey nevi) are a type of flat birthmark that usually affects babies with more melanated, darker skin. These patches of pigment often appear on the thighs, buttocks and back. They should be documented in your baby's notes at birth so that they aren't mistaken for bruises. Blue-grey spots usually disappear within a couple of years, although some can stick around for much longer. Another type of birthmark is the 'stork bite' or nevus simplex: these are pink patches often found at the nape of the neck or forehead. Temporary 'stork bites' occur in about one-third of all newborns, and are due to a stretching of certain blood vessels – they may become darker when the baby cries or the temperature changes.

A common concern parents have is the newborn rash. Your beautiful baby has just been born and you are a couple of weeks into your postnatal journey. You wake up one morning to find their face covered in an angry-looking red rash. It doesn't appear to be bothering them, but what on earth is it?

Toxic erythema of the newborn (also known as erythema toxicum, erythema toxicum neonatorum, milk spots and baby acne) is a common rash seen in newborns. It affects as many as half of all full-term newborn infants, but is less common in infants born prematurely. There is no known cause, although it is thought to be a baby's reaction to heat or the new environment outside of the womb. Tiny spots similar to a heat rash usually appear on the face first, and can sometimes spread to the torso and limbs. Toxic erythema does not cause a baby to be unwell.

Most cases of toxic erythema of the newborn begin in the first few days after birth, although onset can be as late as 2 weeks of age. It can appear quite angry and widespread, but is usually not as bad as it looks. You don't need to put anything on your baby's face to treat it, as the spots will disappear within a few weeks. Rarely, a newborn rash can be a sign of something more serious so it's worthwhile mentioning it to your doctor or midwife, especially if you are concerned about other symptoms.

Newborn baby skin is 30 per cent thinner than adults. It loses more moisture in the first 3–4 years so needs to be treated with care. It's advised not to put any lotions, potions or oils on newborn skin for the first month. After that, care should be taken to select mild baby products if you want to use them, with a pH level between 5.5 and 7. Most baby products will be transparent about this on either the packaging or on their website. Ensuring frequent nappy changes and keeping skin dry will also help to protect from nappy rash.

Baby Hygiene

Knowing how to manage your baby's hygiene may seem a little daunting, especially if you have never handled a newborn before.

Caring for the umbilical cord stump

When the umbilical cord is clamped and cut, the tissue that is left will start to die off. There are no nerves in the cord, so cutting it isn't painful for you or the baby.

Anything from 5 to 15 days after your baby is born, the umbilical stump will dry out, turn black and drop off. After the stump comes off, it usually takes a further 7 to 10 days for the belly button to heal completely, and your baby may have a slight 'outie' belly button for a few months before it flattens.

Until the stump drops off and the belly button is completely healed, it's important to keep the area clean and dry, to prevent infection. Here is some general guidance on caring for the umbilical cord stump:

- If you bathe baby before the stump falls off, ensure you pat dry around the stump properly after.
- Use cotton wool or a cotton bud and cooled boiled water to clean gently around the stump each day. There is no evidence to show powders or any other lotions and potions help to heal the area quicker or prevent infection.
- You may notice a slight smell as the stump turns black, which is normal. If the smell becomes overpowering, however, you may want to seek advice from your GP or midwife.
- As the stump heals, it may look a little oozy, especially if accidentally knocked. You may also notice brown/yellow stains on baby's clothing on occasion. If the discharge is persistent, blood-stained or really odorous, seek advice from your GP or midwife.
- Roll the nappy under the stump or have it covering it, to avoid it rubbing and irritating your baby's skin.
- Occasionally the area can become infected, but this is not common. The main sign is inflamed red skin on the area of the abdomen around the stump and/or a temperature of 37.6°C or more. Inform your midwife or GP if you notice this.
- Keeping the area clean and dry as well as minimal touching will help promote natural drying and healing.

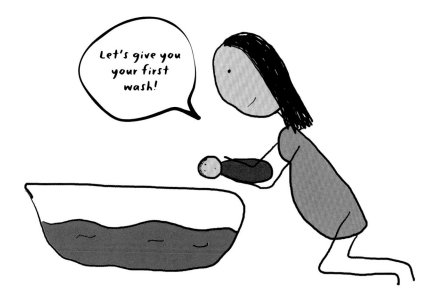

Bathing baby

The vernix substance I mentioned on page 222 has amazing moisturising and antibacterial properties. It is better to rub it into the skin than wash it off, and there is no need to wash your baby straight after the birth. Many parents wait a few days before bathing their baby and decide not to bathe every day. You may prefer to wash their face, neck, hands and genital/bottom area through 'top and tailing' instead of bathing them. Top and tailing just requires a bowl of warm water and cotton wool. Get everything you need ready before you start, including a towel, a fresh nappy and clean clothes. Here is a step-by-step guide to top and tailing:

1. Ensure you are in a warm room, undress baby on a clean towel or changing mat, and wrap them in a towel, allowing their head and neck to be exposed. Leave the nappy on for now.
2. Dip the cotton wool in the water without drenching it and wipe gently around your baby's eyes, from the nose outward. Use a separate piece of cotton wool for each eye. This avoids cross-contamination if your baby happens to have an eye infection (this is fairly common in newborns).
3. Use a clean piece of cotton wool for each ear, but never push inside or use cotton buds to clean inside the ears. This is not necessary and may cause infection and/or damage to the inner ear. Wash the rest of your baby's face, neck and hands and dry them gently with the towel.
4. Remove your baby's nappy and wash their genital area and bottom using separate cotton wool for each part. Dry very carefully, making sure the skin is dry between the skin folds, and put on a clean nappy. Be sure to dress baby quickly to avoid them getting cold.

When you are ready to give baby a full bath, you might prefer to use a small baby bath or large washing-up-sized bowl to begin with, especially if you have never bathed a baby before: babies can be quite slippery, and trying to lean into a full-sized bath first time around can be daunting for any new parent! As with the 'top and tailing', ensure you have everything you need to hand prior to starting, and that the room is warm:

1. Fill the baby bath or bowl to around 10cm and test the temperature by dipping your elbow in (your elbow is more sensitive than your fingers). The water should be warm to the touch – warm enough so as not to turn cold after five minutes.

2. You do not need to add bathing products or bubbles to the water for at least the first month.

3. It's best not to bathe your baby straight after a feed as they may get uncomfortable or vomit.

4. Holding your baby on your knee, clean their face as you would if top and tailing.

5. Wash their hair with plain water, supporting them over the bowl.

6. Gently dry the hair, take off baby's nappy and clean their bottom if needed.

7. Lower your baby gently into the baby bath or bowl, using one hand to support them under their shoulders. The baby's head should be rested on your arm while doing this.

8. Keep your baby's head clear of the water and use the other hand to gently wash the water over your baby's body.

9. Never leave your baby alone in the bath, not even for a second.

10. Once washed, after a few minutes, lift your baby out and gently pat them dry, making sure all of the creases and folds are no longer damp.

Bathing can be a great way for both parents to have bonding time with the baby, especially if mum is breastfeeding.

Nappy changing

After the first week, you will find that you change quite a few nappies per day, sometimes up to twelve in twenty-four hours! Changing nappies often will help to prevent nappy rash which affects up to a third of babies and toddlers in nappies at any one time.

Babies need changing as soon as possible when they have done a poo, to prevent nappy rash. Only change night-time nappies if you know your baby has pooped or the nappy feels very full, as this is likely to leak and cause discomfort. If the nappy is just slightly wet from urine, it is okay to let them sleep. Good-quality nappies are super absorbent so it's likely that a little of urine won't be in direct contact with the skin for long periods. Whether you choose disposable or reusable nappies is totally up to you. Disposable nappies can be discarded with general waste. Reusable nappies require liners which catch the majority of any mess. Washing them on a hot 60°C wash will destroy most bacteria present.

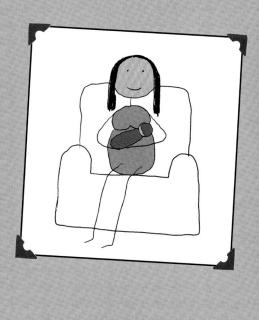

As babies grow and their stomachs become capable of holding more milk, the time between feeds often stretches as they can take more at each feed.

Jaundice

Jaundice is a condition that can affect anyone of any age. It's more common to see it in newborns as opposed to adults, primarily because a newborn's liver is immature and therefore needs to work harder than an adult's.

Jaundice occurs when there is too much of a substance called bilirubin in the blood (a yellow waste product of red blood cells) and the liver is unable to remove it quickly enough. This can make the skin and eyes appear yellow, signalling jaundice.

There are several indicators which may suggest your baby has jaundice, including yellowing of the skin, which is easier to identify in lighter-skinned babies, bright yellow urine, yellow whites of the eyes, soles of feet and palms of hands and yellowing of gums. If your baby has dark skin, you may be able to identify yellowing by pressing gently on the tip of your baby's nose. Some of these signs are subtle, while others are obvious. A very obviously jaundiced baby may need a blood test to check how high the bilirubin levels are. If the levels are high, your baby may need to be treated with a UV lamp to help clear the jaundice. In rare cases, the bilirubin levels are high enough to warrant a blood transfusion.

A very jaundiced baby may be really sleepy and difficult to wake for feeds. If you suspect jaundice, be sure to raise your concerns with your care provider during your postnatal care.

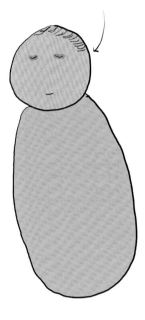

Yellowing of skin and eyes

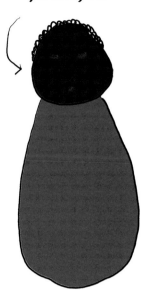

In darker skin tones, yellowing of eyes and under tongue/gums. Gently pressing tip of nose may show yellowing too

There are two types of jaundice in newborns: **physiological** and **pathological**.

/ **PHYSIOLOGICAL JAUNDICE** usually occurs around 3 days after the baby is born and causes a mild yellowing of the skin. You may hear of the term 'breastmilk jaundice' from relatives or friends – this is it! It's fairly common in (though not exclusive to) breastfed babies and usually resolves itself after a couple of weeks, with lots of feeding: keeping baby hydrated is key. Physiological jaundice is very common – it's estimated that over 50 per cent of babies will develop some degree of it. Occasionally it can go on for longer than a couple of weeks, sometimes resulting in additional monitoring from midwives and doctors on an outpatient basis.

/ **PATHOLOGICAL JAUNDICE** is highly irregular and can occur within twenty-four hours of birth, causing severely high bilirubin levels. This extremely rare type of jaundice may be caused by liver or blood disorders and is much more concerning. If an extremely high level of bilirubin builds up it can cause bilirubin toxicity, which can have cause complications with the baby.

Screening Tests

We are fortunate in the UK to have a newborn screening service available on the NHS which includes checking hearing, and screening blood for a variety of rare disorders.

Hearing test

Although hearing loss in newborns is rare, affecting around 1–2 in 1,000, babies who have hearing loss diagnosed from birth can be treated and supported immediately, giving them a better chance to develop language, speech and communication skills. These skills will help them to thrive through relationships with family or carers from an early age.

Most babies who suffer permanent hearing loss have no history of it in their families. Babies who are extremely premature, and those who have serious medical needs, are more likely to suffer from hearing problems.

If you have your baby in a hospital, chances are you will be offered a screening test for hearing before you go home. You may miss this opportunity if you have an early discharge but it's okay – an appointment can be made for you to return to hospital, or at another clinical community setting, at a later stage. The local newborn hearing screening service will contact you to arrange a suitable time and place for the screening to go ahead.

The screening test takes only a few minutes. A tiny earpiece is placed in your baby's ear, usually when they are asleep, and a series of clicking sounds are made. Responses from the ear are recorded but clear responses aren't always obtained. Quite often, babies have to have a second test if the baby is unsettled at the time of the original one, if there is fluid in the ear, or if there is a lot of background noise.

This hearing check is very good at detecting hearing problems and will not cause your baby any harm.

Blood spot test

This screening test – the newborn blood spot test (NBBS) – is done when the baby is around 5 days old. This test involves taking a blood sample from your baby's foot using a small device and putting five drops onto a special sheet of paper. It is then sent off to a laboratory to find out if the baby has any of a number of rare but serious health conditions. Most babies will not have any, but if something is picked up, the benefits of knowing early for these babies is huge. Early treatment can improve their health and prevent severe disability and complications further down the line.

The test is usually carried out by a midwife either at home or in a postnatal clinic. The conditions that it looks for are:

- Sickle cell disease, which affects 1 in 2,000 babies in the UK.
- Cystic fibrosis, which affects 1 in 2,500 babies in the UK.
- Congenital hypothyroidism, which affects 1 in 3,000 babies in the UK.
- Inherited metabolic disorders – phenylketonuria (PKU), medium-chain acyl-CoA dehydrogenase deficiency (MCADD), maple syrup urine disease (MSUD), isovaleric acidaemia (IVA), glutaric aciduria type 1 (GA1), homocystinuria (pyridoxine unresponsive) (HCU).

Approximately 1 in 10,000 babies in the UK have PKU or MCADD. The other metabolic disorders are even rarer, affecting around 1 in 100,000 to 1 in 150,000 babies.

The results are given to you by a health professional, by the time your baby is 6–8 weeks old.

Coping With A Baby And A Small Child/Children

If this is not your first baby, you may be wondering how you'll manage, particularly if the age gap between your children is close.

One of the things I was dreading when pregnant with my last baby was how I would manage caring for my then two-year-old as well. He was (and still is) very high maintenance, and splitting my time between them both seemed impossible. Having had twins as well, I can safely say that looking after two babies was nothing compared to having a toddler running riot and a baby too. At the hospital, my son was in awe of his sister but when it came to taking her home, he wasn't too impressed! There was a massive fight for my attention when I was breastfeeding her, as he hadn't long stopped breastfeeding himself and he wanted to give it a go again. Having support from their dad was paramount – the 2 weeks' paternity leave really helped as he could distract our son and play with him when I was caught up with the baby.

It can be tough, but some things I found that helped were:

- Encouraging the older one to help with fetching nappies, clothes etc.
- Bathing them together.
- Wearing the baby in a sling to enable free hands! (My baby didn't like to be put down for long.)
- Eventually as baby got bigger I tried to make them nap at the same time. Wearing them both out through play and stimulation beforehand may help with this.
- Having a bag of snacks and/or activities ready so that the eldest could entertain himself when I was preoccupied with the baby.
- Asking for help at times when it became too much.
- Taking a drive out to local shops in the evening when Dad was home, to get five minutes to myself and buy chocolate!

Most importantly, I reminded myself that I was doing a great job even when I didn't always feel like it. If you have a toddler and are expecting a baby, you will be pretty busy for a while, but they grow so fast and the bond that siblings have can be amazing!

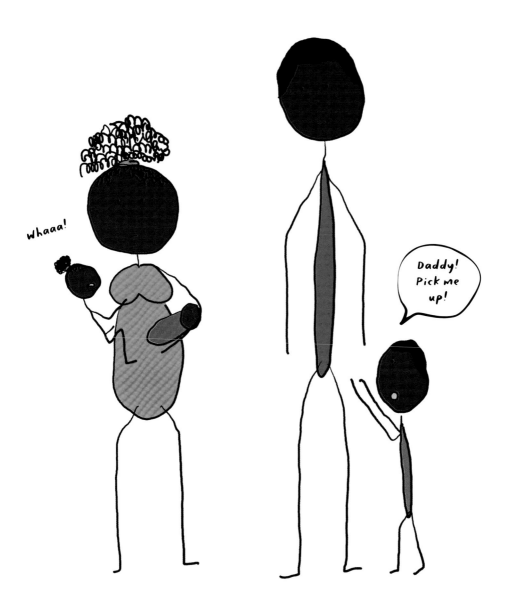

Partners And Bonding

Many partners worry that they may not get the opportunity to bond with the baby in the same way that the birthing mother has. This is a totally natural feeling, especially if the pregnancy and impending arrival hasn't felt real until the time of birth!

There may be moments when your partner feels a little side-lined, particularly when everything seems to be focused on you and the baby. The main thing to remember is that, as parents, you are both on a journey; a journey to develop a deep and meaningful connection with your child. It's a connection that may not happen instantly, but one that will strengthen over the initial days, weeks and months of your baby's life.

It is normal for newborns to cry a lot when put down, and for them to want to be close to and attached to Mum if breastfeeding. This doesn't mean there aren't ways that partners can bond with baby, too. There is a common misconception that partners struggle to bond if the baby is breastfed – this is simply not true.

The early days can be tough, but having patience and working together as a team will go a long way. Babies will benefit from both parents offering lots of skin-to-skin contact, cuddles and closeness. It also helps with their brain development and, over time, babies will have unconditional love for both parents.

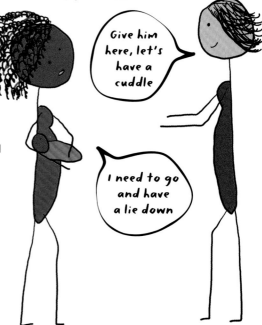

I asked a variety of new, non-birthing parents how they bonded with their baby. Here is what they said:

'I bathed the baby, that was our time to bond and also gave my partner a chance to rest.'

'At night-time, I used to try and settle the baby after she was breastfed. It worked a treat.'

'I would try and be as hands-on as possible, changing nappies and getting involved with bath time.'

'Reading him a story was our thing.'

'I didn't realise skin to skin was something for dads until the midwife suggested it after he was born. From that day on, we did it all the time.'

'I carry my son around in a sling. I think he likes the sound of my heart beating as he is always really chilled.'

'Apparently I'm the playful one. My little girl has always enjoyed playtime with me. I witnessed her first laugh when we were exploring lights and shapes on the baby gym.'

'My wife got me involved in a baby massage course. I found it a great way to settle my daughter.'

'Bedtime routine, including a story and lots of cuddles.'

'Burping her after she fed and taking her for short walks, just me and her.'

Babies And Sleep

In the early days and weeks after your baby is born, it's unlikely that you will have any kind of set routine to your day.

In those first few days and weeks, your baby will require responsive feeding – they show cues that they are hungry (which you will learn to recognise), and you feed them. This will be accompanied with a sleep pattern that is very unpredictable. Newborns usually have very short sleep cycles, which cause them to wake often throughout the day and night.

One of the biggest concerns I have heard from new mothers is that baby sleeps a lot during the day but is awake most of night. This is totally normal! Think back to pregnancy: you probably spent much of the day busy, moving around, rocking baby to sleep. At night-time, you may have noticed that baby wakes up when you're in bed, kicking and letting you know that they're there with increased activity. This pattern will continue after birth. Along with the fact that prolactin, the hormone required to make breastmilk, is produced in higher quantities at night-time, it's no wonder that night-time for newborns can often mean anything but sleep! You will probably find that, from 6–8 weeks, patterns will start to emerge naturally and you might want to think about introducing a routine then.

If you are keen to get into a routine from the start, that's okay, just understand that there are limitations to what a newborn baby is and isn't capable of doing. Activities such as bathing them at the same time each evening, followed by quiet time, can help initiate the idea that bedtime is approaching. Whether you are breast or formula feeding, you will be feeding your baby regularly on a twenty-four-hour clock. Most newborns won't go for longer than a couple of hours in between feeds, though some will be shorter, some longer. The fact that it is night-time makes no difference, but as they grow and their stomachs become capable of holding more milk, the time between feeds often stretches as they can take more at each feed (these longer breaks are usually very welcome at night-time).

When your baby wakes at night for a feed, tend to them quickly and quietly with little fuss, lights or noise. There's no need to wake your baby up for a night feed if they are healthy, gaining weight and there are no concerns such as jaundice (where you may be advised to feed them more often). Your baby will usually let you know when they are hungry. If they allow you a couple of extra hours' sleep, accept it!

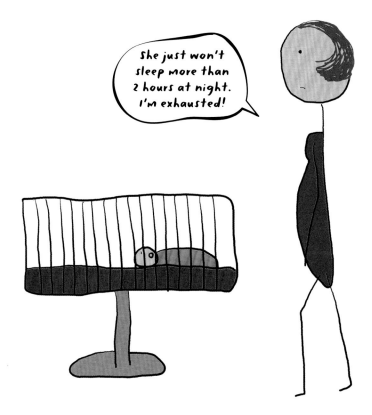

Safe sleep

Knowing how to safely put your baby down to sleep will help them to remain comfortable, get a restful sleep and reduce the risk of SIDS (sudden infant death syndrome). SIDS is the sudden and unexpected death of a baby under 1 year old. Although it sounds distressing, it's important to point out that SIDS is rare, affecting around 200 babies every year in the UK. Here are the guidelines for promoting safe sleep:

- Keep your baby in your bedroom to sleep for at least the first 6 months.
- Your baby should have their own space to sleep, i.e. a basket or crib, away from any radiators.
- Put your baby to sleep in a sleep bag or, if you don't have one, just one blanket. Avoid multiple blankets, soft toys and crib bumpers. Overheating and suffocation are simple to avoid by keeping the sleeping space clear.
- Put baby to sleep on their back with their feet at the bottom of the cot or crib. Once they get to an age where they can roll, you can allow them to adopt a sleeping position that is more comfortable for them.

- Use a new, firm mattress for them to sleep on.
- Never fall asleep with your baby on the sofa or in a chair. There is a chance of baby rolling off and getting wedged between a parent and the chair.
- Don't smoke or allow anyone else to smoke in the same house as your baby, or around them at all. Anyone who smokes should wash their hands before touching your baby.
- If you decide you want to swaddle your baby, do it safely. Ensure the wrap is made of thin, breathable material, never swaddle too tight or above the shoulders. The baby's knees should still be able to bend up. Never ever place a swaddled baby on their front.
- Breastfeed if you are able to. Research has shown that breastfeeding exclusively for 2 months reduces the risk of SIDS by 50 per cent and at 6 months, it's reduced by over 60 per cent.

So, what about bed sharing or co-sleeping? This is quite a controversial topic, as we know that many parents do bed share with their babies – we all want a restful sleep, right? Although the advice is to not sleep in the same bed as your baby, there are some parents who choose to do so, especially when struggling with a baby who wants to always be close to them!

If you decide to bed share, here are some guidelines given by The Lullaby Trust to ensure you do it as safely as possible:

- Make sure the area of the bed that baby sleeps in is cleared of pillows and bedding.
- Avoid placing the baby between you and your partner.
- Place them on their back to sleep.
- Never leave them in or on an adult bed alone.
- Do not bed share if any adults in the bed have consumed alcohol, or drugs that cause drowsiness, or smoke.

It can be dangerous to bed share if your newborn was premature or of low birth weight (less than 2.5kg).

Caring For Twins Or More

Caring for one baby can be hard work. Caring for two or more can be extremely stressful, especially in the early days.

The biggest worry for most people expecting multiples isn't necessarily the birth, but caring for them once they are here. There may be financial concerns, concerns about support, sleeping, feeding and even sharing the love between them. All of these concerns are normal and valid when you are expecting more than one baby.

Every journey with having multiples will be different. The majority of multiples are born before their estimated due date for a variety of reasons. These babies will often have a stay in the neonatal intensive care unit (NICU), but many will be born close to full term and will go home from the hospital with their parents.

The first thing you'll want to ensure when you know you're expecting more than one baby is that you have an adequate supply of everything. This includes nappies, clothing, bedding and washing powder. If you have a good support network of friends and family, discuss with them how they can help you in the early days, whether that be coming over to simply offer a pair of hands to hold one of the babies so you can deal with the other, or so that either you or your partner can have a much-needed break. I remember finding simple things difficult, such as having a shower while they were awake. With my singleton children, I would take them into the bathroom with me in a bouncer so that I could wash while still having them within eyesight. Trying to fit two babies and two bouncers in the bathroom was much trickier. Sharing the load with your partner or family really can make all the difference.

Having more than one baby means more mouths to feed, more crying and more babies to get to sleep. It can become incredibly overwhelming and difficult to cope with if they are doing this at different times. Getting multiple babies into a routine of sorts is important if you want to avoid burn-out. This is somewhat different to my advice on caring for a single newborn and consideration of the fourth trimester, but routine is essential to be able to manage with the load that having more than one newborn entails.

When thinking about routines, do consider that all newborns want to feed on demand. Therefore, if one of your babies appears to be showing signs that they want to feed, offer a feed to the other one(s) as well. If you do this, you will probably notice that in time, they will all get used to feeding together. When I had my twins 14 years ago, I made the mistake of feeding each one 'on demand' when I first brought them home from hospital. Now, while this is the best practice when you have one baby, when you have more than one, you will likely end up spending the whole night constantly feeding one baby or the other. The continuous cycle is exhausting (as I found out, the hard way). After changing the way I did things, I soon got them feeding together, which was better all round for everyone.

If you are breastfeeding, you may want to try tandem feeding – having two babies on a breast each at the same time – or you may feel more comfortable feeding one straight after the other. If you are bottle feeding, anticipate their feeds so that you can start to prepare the bottles in advance of them being hungry. Remember to stick to the safe bottle feeding guidelines on pages 196–197.

Bath times should be a family affair, too. When they are tiny, bathe them one at a time with either you and your partner bathing, drying, dressing a baby each, or one bathing and one drying. If you are bathing your babies alone, have them all close by, perhaps in a bouncer as you bathe each baby one at a time. When they are old enough to sit unaided, you may find it easier to bathe them together.

Ask your health visitor if they know of any local twins/multiples groups, as you may find it useful to share tips and stories with other parents having similar experiences. The Twins Trust (*twinstrust.org*) is another excellent resource that you may find helpful.

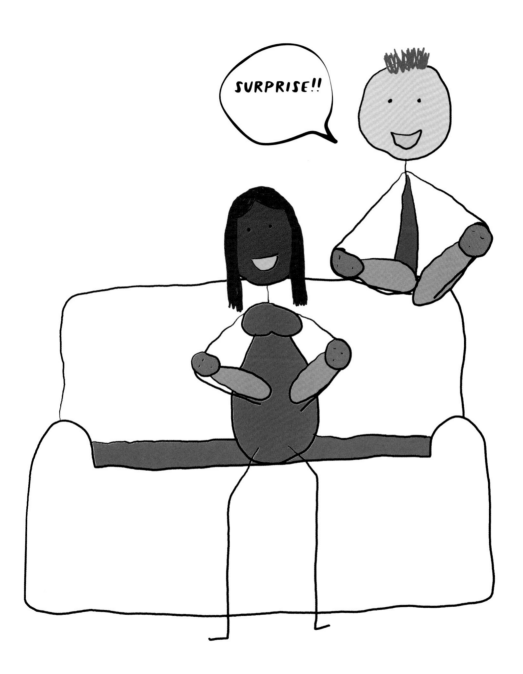

Why Babies Cry

As a new parent, one of the most stressful things is having a baby that cries and you don't know why. Newborn babies cry on average for about two and a half hours each day, on and off. This may seem like a lot but it's their only form of communication. I'm sure there are times when adults spend longer than two and a half hours communicating by talking!

When babies cry they are communicating a need for something. This could be a need for food, a need to be more comfortable (perhaps they are too cold/warm/have a wet nappy), a need for closeness and comfort, a need for sleep if they are over-tired, or they are experiencing pain of some sort. Over time you will figure out what each cry means, but initially you may find yourself going through all of the motions trying to sooth your baby.

Sometimes, babies cry a lot more than expected, over a longer timeframe. If a baby cries continually for three hours or more each day, this is known as colic. Colic (excessive crying) is thought to be caused by intestinal cramping or trapped wind causing abdominal pain. It can be extremely distressing for both the baby and parents when a baby has colic. You may feel helpless, as often babies who suffer from this are inconsolable. Colic does tend to subside by the time a baby is 6 months old, however. If you suspect your baby has colic, reach out to your health visitor or GP for advice. Depending on whether there are other symptoms, i.e. changes in bowel movements, reflux or vomiting, your care provider may make suggestions of food-elimination diets if breastfeeding, changing milk if formula-feeding or may even recommend an anti-colic medication to try.

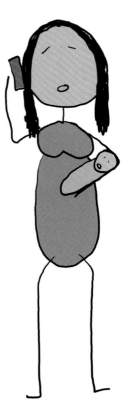

Mum, she just cries ALL day long. What can I do?

There are some things you can try if you find that your baby is crying a lot and you're unsure what to do. During the first few months after birth, mimicking the comfort of the womb may help the baby feel more secure. Dr Harvey Karp wrote a blog post about using the 'Five S's' to calm a baby when they appear inconsolable. I have added an additional two (skin to skin and sling) and adapted it to the 'Seven S's'.

/ **SWADDLING**. Some babies like to be wrapped securely (not tightly) using a light wrap. This prevents them from flailing their arms around and startling themselves.

/ **SHUSHING**. In the womb, the baby will have heard lots of whooshing noises as the maternal blood rushed around the body. By making gentle 'shhhh' sounds to your newborn, you are helping to recreate that environment.

/ **SIDE/STOMACH-LYING**. This is not recommended as a sleeping position, but if your baby has gas or griping pain in the stomach, lying them like this on your lap or a blanket for a short while can help to calm them and also aid with digestion. Many neonatal intensive care units (NICUs) lay babies on their stomachs too for this exact reason. NICU units are constantly attended and babies are monitored around the clock, reducing the risk of SIDS.

/ **SWING**. Gently rocking a baby from side to side, or trying a baby swing if you have one, may help. They were used to that motion in the womb, so of course still want it to continue.

/ **SUCK**. Suckling often calms a baby down. Whether it's a breast, pacifier or bottle, you may find that this is just what they need.

/ **SKIN TO SKIN**. Being skin to skin with your baby is extremely beneficial. It can help promote calm, keep them warm, they can hear your heartbeat and it stimulates the release of the feel-good hormone, oxytocin.

/ **SLING**. Wearing your baby in a sling is another way to calm them down. If you use a baby sling or carrier, follow the UK Sling Consortium's TICK guidelines to prevent accidental asphyxiation or overheating:

- **Tight** – The sling should be tight enough to hold them close.
- **In view at all times** – You should be able to see your baby's face by glancing down, there should be no fabric covering their face.
- **Close enough to kiss** – Your baby's head should be as close to your chin as possible. You should be able to kiss them easily.
- **Keep chin off the chest** – A baby in a sling or carrier should never be so curled up that their chin is sitting on their chest.
- **Supported back** – Your baby's back should be supported in its natural position. The back shouldn't appear bent or unaligned. If the sling is too loose, the baby may potentially slump, closing off their airway.

Give these a go when your baby needs calming – you may be pleasantly surprised!

If Your Baby
Is In The NICU

Some babies will need extra care and support after they are born,
meaning they are transferred to the neonatal intensive care unit (NICU).

Most of the babies that enter the NICU are premature and need help with things like
breathing, as their lungs are underdeveloped. Sometimes full-term babies may go to the
NICU if there are other issues such as persistent low sugar levels, suspected infection
or resuscitation at birth (to name a few).

Some parents are briefed and prepared for what to expect if they know in advance that
their baby will be spending some time in the NICU. Before I gave birth to my twins at
34 weeks, I met the neonatal team who explained the process, and was even shown the
NICU so that I wasn't shocked at all the tiny babies in incubators.

All babies in the NICU require individualised care and have different needs. Some babies,
especially the very tiny preterm babies, will need help breathing for some time and will
have breathing tubes. Some babies may not have the breathing tubes if they are more
stable, but might have feeding tubes in their nose instead, if they are unable to suckle.

There are usually different areas for different levels of care. For example, in my NICU
there was the intensive care area where most babies were in incubators with breathing
apparatus and one-to-one care, and the other area that they graduated to as they grew
and their health improved. This area would see babies in open cots and more hands-on
care from parents.

If your baby goes to the NICU, there a few things to be aware of:

- Hygiene is key. Hands must always be washed on entering the unit.
- Your baby may be fed through a nasal feeding tube if their suckling reflex has not developed.
- If your baby is preterm and unable to suckle directly from the breast, expressing breastmilk is highly recommended. It helps protect their gut from an infection that they are more prone to when born early.
- Don't worry if you are unable to express much in the first couple of days. This is really common and hand expressing may be helpful (see page 190).
- There should be a designated milk pumping room and fridge to store your milk. When pumping at home, you can store it in your fridge and bring it to the NICU when you visit your baby.

Having a baby that has to spend time in the NICU can be a daunting, scary and worrying time. There are lots of organisations that support families experiencing this, including Bliss, Tommy's and the Rainbow Trust. You might also find groups online for parents of babies in the same boat. It may help to talk to others who are in a similar situation to you.

Miscarriage And Stillbirth

Whatever stage you lose a baby, during or after pregnancy, it's devastating. Pregnancy is supposed to be a happy and exciting time and it usually is, but sometimes a pregnancy can end unexpectedly with a miscarriage or stillbirth.

Even though miscarriage is extremely common, affecting an estimated one in eight pregnancies for those who are aware they are pregnant, it doesn't make it any easier to bear. A miscarriage is the loss of a baby at up to 23 weeks of pregnancy and can occur in a multitude of ways. Early miscarriages, up to 12 weeks' gestation, can appear as the following:

- *An ectopic pregnancy* – A pregnancy which doesn't develop in the uterus, often growing in the fallopian tube instead.

- *A chemical pregnancy* – The egg is fertilised but doesn't implant properly in the womb. This can result in a positive pregnancy test, along with symptoms, but on ultrasound there appears to be no gestational sac or placenta.

- *A blighted ovum* – The fertilised egg implants in the lining of the uterus, but only begins to develop a placenta without an embryo.

Sometimes a miscarriage occurs spontaneously, and the cause for this is unknown. Often cramping and bleeding is experienced, followed by expulsion of the baby, a tiny embryo and sac that may or may not be visible, depending on the gestation. If a miscarriage does not occur spontaneously, but it's been discovered on ultrasound that sadly there is no viable pregnancy, a woman may opt to have a procedure called a D & C (dilation and curettage) in hospital, or medication to help to empty the uterus.

A late miscarriage is one that occurs during the second trimester of pregnancy up to 23 weeks and 6 days. A miscarriage experienced later in the pregnancy can be particularly difficult as there likely will have been noticeable physical changes to the body, the baby's movements may have been felt and, if an ultrasound had been performed, there will likely be memories of watching the baby wriggling around on the screen. A late miscarriage can be spontaneous. The uterus begins to cramp, initiating labour, which may or may not be accompanied by bleeding, or it may be detected on an ultrasound with the absence of the baby's heartbeat.

The age of viability for a baby is officially 24 weeks – some babies are born alive earlier than this but will rarely survive. A stillbirth is the loss of a baby after 24 weeks of pregnancy. After months of preparing for the baby, experiencing a stillbirth can be a particularly painfully heartbreaking thing to go through, especially when often a full labour is experienced to birth the baby.

The majority of stillbirths are detected after a woman has noticed the baby's movements have stopped. Stillbirth occurs in approximately 1 in 250 births in the UK and can happen as a result of numerous causes, such as poor growth in the uterus or placental abruption. Occasionally, the cause for a stillbirth is unknown.

If a baby is born alive and then dies within 28 days after birth, it is known as a neonatal death. When a baby dies after birth, it may be expected or unexpected. Either way, it can cause unimaginable heartache. It's natural for parents suffering with such loss to ask questions and to need lots of support in dealing with grief.

How someone copes with a miscarriage or stillbirth at any stage varies enormously. Some people want to talk about their baby often, others would rather initiate conversation when they want to, but would prefer not to have others constantly talking and asking questions. If you experience a miscarriage it's important to give yourself time to grieve the loss in your own time, in your own manner. There should be health professionals available to support you, and bereavement midwives are often available if you have had a late miscarriage or stillbirth. If you have experienced an early miscarriage and haven't yet met a midwife, your GP should be able to signpost support or counselling should you need it.

There are a range of support services and charities that may be beneficial too, such as Tommy's, SANDS and the Miscarriage Association.

Resources

- NHS pregnancy guidance *pnhs.uk/pregnancy*
- Evidence and studies surrounding birth *evidencebasedbirth.com*
- UK maternity leave guidance *gov.uk/employers-maternity-pay-leave*
- Maternity care options in the UK *which.co.uk/reviews/birthing-options*
- Information on independent midwives in the UK *imuk.org.uk*
- Information and advice on twins and multiple births *twinstrust.org*
- Birth rights *birthrights.org.uk*
- Information and support on perinatal mental health *pandasfoundation.org.uk*
- Pregnancy sickness support *pregnancysicknesssupport.org.uk*
- Tommy's charity *tommys.org*
- Miscarriage support *miscarriageassociation.org.uk*
- Stillbirth and neonatal death charity *sands.org.uk*
- *Inducing Labour: making informed decisions*, by Dr Sara Wickham (Birthmoon Creations, 2018)
- *Why Induction Matters*, by Rachel Reed (Pinter & Martin Ltd., 2018)

Hypnobirthing

To find out more about my hypnobirthing course, and how it can help you to have a confident, calm and empowering birth, visit *midwifemarley.com*.

Index

Doppler 137, 143
doulas 162-3
down breathing 128
Down's syndrome 34
drinks to avoid 25, 211
drugs, recreational 27, 67, 159
due dates 12-13, 22, 133

E

early pregnancy units (EPU) 86
ectopic pregnancies 246
eggs 25
emotions: after birth 204-5
  during pregnancy 40-1, 44
'en caul' 120
endorphins 106
Entonox 136, 138, 139-40
environment 97, 106, 130
epidurals 97, 104, 110, 112, 127, 140-1, 143, 148
epigastric (chest) pain 87
episiotomy 80, 103, 114, 146
exercise 26-7, 58, 59, 80, 95, 212-13
external cephalic version (ECV) 154

F

fatigue 21, 59
feeding equipment 89
feeding times 227
fibroids 51, 157
first trimester 21
fish, oily 25
fitness 95
fluid retention 63-4
foetus: foetal distress 116
  foetal movements 21, 67, 68-9, 87, 116, 134, 143, 247
  foetal positions 71-3
  IUGR (intrauterine growth restriction) 67, 84
foley balloon 134
folic acid 23
fontanelle 194
food: cooking in advance 88
  cravings 24
  diet and supplements 23-4, 210-11
  food aversions 21
  food poisoning 25
  food to avoid or consume with caution 25, 211
forceps 104, 127, 141, 145, 146
forewaters 122
formula feeding 196-7, 240
fourth trimester 168-247
fundal height 16, 45

G

gas and air see Entonox
gender 21, 103

genetics 95
gestation 12, 36
gestational diabetes 19, 32, 64-5, 67, 84, 134
glucose tolerance test (GTT) 32, 65
golden hour 172-3, 187
Group B Streptococcus (GBS) 78

H

haemorrhage 112
  antenatal (APH) 66-7
  postpartum (PPH) 37, 51, 112, 156-7, 202, 207
haemorrhoids 53, 58, 60
hair: during pregnancy 38-9, 214
  postnatal changes 214-15
headaches 54, 87
health visitors 200
healthy pregnancies 23-7, 95
hearing test 230
heart palpitations 56
heart rate: baby's 16, 143, 144, 221
  mother's 85
heartburn 62
high blood pressure 19, 51, 63, 65, 67, 84, 157, 207
hindwaters 122
home: going home from hospital 180-1
  leaving the house 216-18
homebirths 102, 104, 106, 136, 139-40, 152, 167
hormones see individual hormones
hospital births 104, 106
  going home after 180-1
  support in 176-7
  when to go to 115-17
hydration 24, 31, 53, 54, 57, 60, 70, 210
hygiene, baby 224-6
Hyperemesis gravidarum (HG) 31
hypertension 19, 51, 63, 65, 67, 84, 157, 207
hypnobirthing 83, 116, 124, 128, 138, 139

I

ICP (intrahepatic cholestasis of pregnancy) 86, 134
illness in babies 220-1
implantation bleeding 28
incontinence 114
indigestion 62
induction 97, 132, 133-5, 136, 143
infections 122
instrumental delivery 104
insulin 64
intervention 95, 97, 100, 133
iron 24, 58, 62, 113
itching 87, 141
IUGR (intrauterine growth restriction) 67, 84, 134, 143
IVF (in vitro fertilisation) 13, 74

shows 115
SIDS (sudden infant death syndrome) 237-8
6-week check 200
skin: baby's 222-3
  mother's 38-9, 87
skin-to-skin contact 103, 151, 172-3, 174, 187, 188, 234, 235, 243
sleep 42-3, 54
  babies and 236-8, 243
  during pregnancy 48
  postpartum 180
sleeping accessories 89
slings 183, 235, 243
smell, sense of 21
smoking 27, 67, 159
smoothie, date 81
spider veins 58
spina bifida 23
spots 38
spotting 28-9, 66, 87
statutory maternity pay (SMP) 76
sterilising bottles 197
stillbirths 25, 41, 133, 246-7
stools 195
stress 56, 81-3
stretch marks 87
suckling 243
supplements 23, 58
support, postpartum 176-7
swaddling 243
swelling 56-7, 63-4, 80, 87
symphysis pubis dysfunction 60

T
temperature, as sign of illness 221
TENS machine 139
third trimester 21
toddlers: breastfeeding while pregnant 50
  coping with a new baby and 232-3
  pregnancy with a 48-9
  preparing for a new arrival 49
tongue ties 187
top and tailing 225, 226
toxic erythema 222-3
transfusions 37
transition phase 107, 109-11, 128
trimesters 20-1
  see also fourth trimester
twins 45, 67, 74-5, 84, 143, 157, 159, 239-41

U
ultrasound scans 13, 16, 34-6, 45, 67, 74, 76
umbilical cord: abnormalities 67
  caring for the stump 224
  cord prolapse 155
  cutting 103, 112, 150

optimal cord clamping (OCC) 103, 112, 113, 150
up breathing 128
uterus: afterpains 178
  Braxton Hicks 70
  in labour 107, 108, 138
  post birth 112
  round ligament pain 56
  shape of 95
  uterine rupture 152, 153

V
vagina: tears 111, 114, 156
  vaginal birth after caesarean (VBAC) 147, 152-3
  vaginal examinations 124-5, 134
varicose veins 58-9
ventouse 145-6
vernix 222, 225
visitors 198-9
visual disturbances 87
vitamins 23
  vitamin A 23
  vitamin D 211
vomiting 30-1, 87

W
walking 80, 119, 212
water 24
water births 105, 126, 136-7, 138
waters, breaking 97, 115, 116, 120-2, 155
weight (baby) 194-5, 200
weight (mother): weight gain 46-7
  weight loss 210
work 76-7

Y
yoga 55, 72, 80, 212

Acknowledgements

It has been a dream of mine to write a book for as long as I can remember. It wouldn't have been possible without the immense support of my agent Megan Staunton, who cheered me on all the way, the dedication of my publishing editor Xa Shaw Stewart and the rest of the Bloomsbury team, and the talented Laura Nickoll and Nikki Dupin from Studio Nic&Lou who magically turned hundreds of pages of black and white text and images into a beautifully formatted, colourful masterpiece.

Thank you, Kicki Hansard, for your awesome contribution on doulas, and thanks also to the midwifery colleagues who have supported and inspired me – Sheena Byron, Louise Broadbridge and Illiyin Morrison, you have all taught me so much.

Thanks too to the past, present and future mums and dads that follow me on social media – I truly appreciate your support, and thank you for sharing your personal stories with me.

Finally, thanks to all the families that I have had the privilege to assist in bringing their babies into the world. A large portion of the knowledge I have accumulated over the years of midwifery has come from these experiences, many of which will be etched in my mind forever.

BLOOMSBURY PUBLISHING
Bloomsbury Publishing Plc
50 Bedford Square, London, WC1B 3DP, UK
29 Earlsfort Terrace, Dublin 2, Ireland

BLOOMSBURY, BLOOMSBURY PUBLISHING and the Diana logo are trademarks
of Bloomsbury Publishing Plc

First published in Great Britain 2022

The information contained in this book is provided by way of general guidance in relation to the
specific subject matters addressed herein, but it is not a substitute for specialist medical advice.
It should not be relied on for medical, health-care, pharmaceutical or other professional advice on
specific health needs. The reader should consult a competent medical or health professional before
adopting any of the suggestions in this book or drawing inferences from it

The author and publisher specifically disclaim, as far as the law allows, any responsibility from any
liability, loss or risk (personal or otherwise) which is incurred as a consequence, directly or indirectly,
of the use and applications of any of the contents of this book

A catalogue record for this book is available from the British Library

ISBN: TPB: 978-1-5266-3939-4; eBook: 978-1-5266-3937-0

10 9 8 7 6 5 4 3 2 1

Project Editor: Laura Nickoll
Designer: Nikki Dupin, Studio Nic&Lou
Indexer: Vanessa Bird

Printed and bound in China by C&C Offset Printing Co, Ltd.

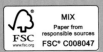

To find out more about our authors and books visit www.bloomsbury.com and sign up for our
newsletters